BACK TO
NATURAL
EATING

Recipes by Emily Jane's Foods

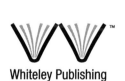

Whiteley Publishing

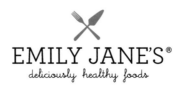

EMILY JANE'S®

deliciously healthy foods

Food photography by Emily Jane Whiteley

Design by RT Design www.rt-design.co.uk

Published by Whiteley Publishing Ltd

First hard cover edition 2011

978-1-908586-70-4

natural

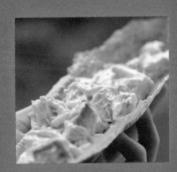

grain free

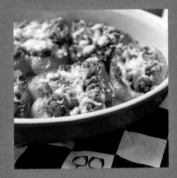

lower carbohydrate

naturally gluten free

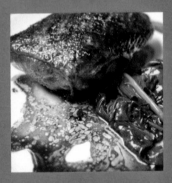

primal-esque

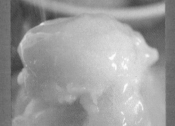

contents

dedication

To my mum, who holds my utmost respect for a never-ending love of life and family despite the odds always seeming to work against her and without whose ruthless determination in the pursuit of health, I would not possess half the health and happiness I have today. x

acknowledgements

Once again for my mum for her endless supply of love, encouragement, strength, support and the frequent loaning of her taste buds!

My dad for being a surprising voice of reason, finding solutions when a way forward seemed impossible, believing in my work and backing me all the way.

My sisters Alice and Lucy for providing a source of endless entertainment.

George, I can't say enough. For being a source of strength and love, even if that does mean forcing me to take some time out occasionally.

My friends for their enthusiastic support, interest and loyalty.

foreword

"At last attention is being paid to the importance of what we eat in our daily diet and its effect on all the systems which contribute to making our bodies work efficiently.

In recent years there has been a slide away from healthy diets with a good combination of protein, carbohydrates in the form of vegetables and fruit and good fats in proper meals. These have been replaced by high carbohydrate and sugar-loaded meals at random times resulting in excessive stimulation of insulin which not only strains the pancreas but also makes our body tissues more resistant to the effect of insulin resulting in myriad symptoms and health problems. Trying to reverse this slide presents challenges, not least because of changed expectations where 'rare' sweet treats become almost a daily and repeated occurrence.

Emily Whiteley has cleverly harnessed this change in demand with the need to ensure a more healthy approach, incorporating more low GI and high protein foods whilst catering to modern tastes. This helps us to think carefully about what we eat and the impact it has on our bodies and, importantly, helps to promote long term health changes in people experiencing symptoms and health conditions which are mystifying them and not responding to normal treatment.

I can highly recommend this series of recipes which takes us, in tandem, along a journey of nutritional education. The long term implications of not heeding this message include well recognised illnesses such as diabetes, heart disease and dementia as well as obesity and it is important for all of us to learn how to incorporate healthy eating in our day-to-day lives so that it becomes a habit not a chore."

To find out more about Miss Sovra Whitcroft and The Surrey Park Clinic you can visit the following website; http://www.thesurreyparkclinic.co.uk/

Sovra Whitcroft MBCHB.FRCOG

Sovra is a consultant gynaecologist who specializes in hormone disorders including Polycystic Ovaries, PMT, Post Natal Depression and menopausal problems. She introduced the concept of treating underlying insulin resistance in parallel with the manipulation and tailoring of female hormones. She runs the Surrey Park Clinic in Guildford which receives referrals from all over the UK because of this approach and because of the increased acceptance that insulin resistance and associated long term health problems are on the increase. The clinic emphasizes the key importance of adjusting diet at the same time as treating with medication and has published on this. She sits on the advisory board of the British Menopause Society.

I am thrilled that Miss Whitcroft agreed to write a foreword to champion this book.

5

introduction

After years of watching the health of my family and myself deteriorate, I quickly understood how incredibly important health is. Wanting to do as much as possible to gain an improved quality of life, giving myself the best chance of recovery, I started to take a closer look at health and diets. Article after article there seemed to be an overwhelming consensus that made sense. More and more articles touted the negative effects of refined sugar and processed carbohydrates (mainly in the form of grains) and negated the villianisation of fats.

Food has become a central part of our social and cultural lives. The 'food is fuel' mentality has become lost and foods are no longer considered on the basis of their nutritional content and quality but instead whether or not they will satisfy our sweet tooth.

A large part of what makes eating healthily so difficult involves social eating. The ability food has to bond people is staggering. Offering a chocolate can give us an excuse to introduce ourselves, inviting new people into our lives. Cooking for another can be a romantic gesture and something as simple as sharing a meal can cement a friendship. However, attempting to eat healthily can become a bit of an issue when eating in company. That awkward feeling begins to arise when a slice of cake is offered, the

inner turmoil and guilt which results, trying to attempt to refuse the offending dish politely without branding yourself a difficult guest. Eventually it becomes too difficult and deciding it's not worth it to irritate the host, we gratefully receive our dish with a nervous smile and dig into the heaving plate. In the rare case we find ourselves able to decline, we feel left out.

Convenience now plays an inevitable role in our hectic lives. Constantly on the go, fitting in eating around our daily events by grabbing something at a supermarket, a sneaky sweet fix from the box of chocolates at work, picking at food whenever possible, not paying as much attention to what or indeed how much we eat as maybe we should. Conversely, eating while considering allergies and intolerances can be intolerable (excuse the pun). Constantly having to be on the alert, thinking about the effect that bite of cake will have on you can just be an unwelcome irritation in life, to say the very least.

Considering all these factors influence the way we eat, it can be difficult to eat healthily. And this is where this book comes in.

This book is an accumulation of the recipes I have developed, after much trial and error and countless dishes pushed under the noses of my poor family and friends for taste testing. When in the process of experimenting with my diet, and ultimately my lifestyle, I wanted to include, not only staple everyday foods which I could happily eat, safe in the knowledge I wouldn't suffer post-meal but the more decadent, special occasion foods I would enjoy and feel happy to share with friends and family. I wanted to veer adamantly away from the notion that healthy, natural foods were a tasteless option only for people with health problems. If I've found anything to be true, it is prevention is always better than cure. Adopting healthier eating patterns, might mean we avoid so many more health problems later in life.

I wanted to write this book to give people back a taste of what they've been missing out on and provide some different foodie ideas. Providing delicious meals, showing that grains and sugar can become a less prevalent part of our food intake. By providing nutritious, tasty alternatives to the unhealthier foods we used to feast on, once again we can happily indulge in some of our old favourites.

Much love,
Emily Jane x

7

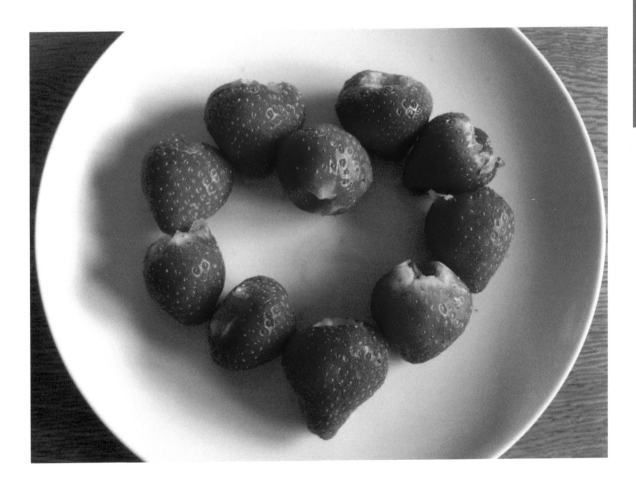

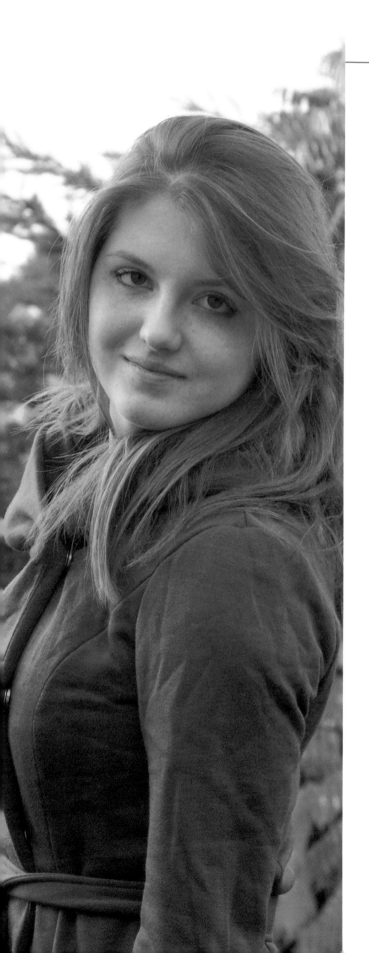

my story

My family…

…has a long history of ill health and from a young age I found myself on the slippery slope that is chronic disease. My mother was unwell with Lyme disease before I was born. Along with her brother, they were both misdiagnosed with M.E. (Myalgic Encephalitis). At the beginning I was less aware of the disease and growing up it became a fact of life that my mum couldn't do certain things that other people could. She drove me to school; walked to the shops; nothing seemed extraordinarily out of place. Then gradually bit by bit, life started changing. Soon my Dziadek (grandfather) took my mums place taking me to school as she became unable to drive and would tire more easily.

A few years later, my story began…

… My first obvious symptoms appearing from age 9, began with bladder and bowel problems. I suffered bouts of depression and my OCD (obsessive compulsive disorder) accelerated. I took medications for the next few years, trying to manage my symptoms.

Feeling in control of the situation and more confident, at age 15 I decided to visit some friends in Germany for a week in my summer holidays. Whilst there I was bitten by a tick and contracted Lyme disease. From that point on my health started to deteriorate with increasing speed. Over the next few years, more symptoms started appearing. I started to become tired easily, with depression and OCD making frequent appearances. I was constantly having sick days off school and when I did make it in, focus and concentration escaped me and my grades suffered tremendously.

Before I knew it, my GCSEs were fast approaching, with revision well under way, I had to work hard to catch up on all the school work missed whilst off sick. Arriving at my 16th birthday I noticed a large weight gain. Desperate to lose the weight, I cut out fats and some refined sugar from my diet and started taking supplements, determined to be in the best of health for my exams.

The first week of my GCSEs flew by. I geared myself up for a truck load of revision over the weekend in preparation for the second week. However in place of the textbooks and assorted practice papers, I found myself between hospitals, having scans and blood tests. It began to sink in that hard-core revision wasn't appearing a likely prospect. In a huge amount of pain, not knowing what was happening, I kept thinking of my exams starting the next morning and the revision I needed to be doing. However I needn't have given the revision a second thought as I didn't make it in for the second week of exams. Instead I acquired a PCOS (polycystic ovarian syndrome) diagnosis and underwent emergency surgery to remove a large torted ovarian cyst.

After a summer, spent relaxing and trying to recover fully, I entered sixth form, ready and raring to put ill health behind me and embark on my new healthy life. Now age 17, I spent half my lower sixth life in hospital or at home. I missed large chunks of school, piling in extra lessons to try to catch up. I

contracted recurrent acute tonsillitis. Every week I'd feel a sinking disappointment as yet again it would return, signalling another course of antibiotics. With a new diagnosis of IBS to add to my repertoire, I became increasingly constipated, bloated and with bouts of intense pain.

Unable to continue constantly high antibiotic doses, I resorted to a tonsillectomy in the Easter holidays before my AS levels. However, little did I know, apparently tonsils are not necessary to contract tonsillitis or at least nobody had informed my throat. So my throat seemed to ignore my attempts to eliminate infection, obstinately allowing the infection/ antibiotics cycle to continue.

My health was slipping away and running out of options, I felt powerless. The day of my last biology AS exam came and my body decided enough was enough. As soon as my paper was taken from me, dizziness took over, forcefully encouraging me to lie down immediately. Holding onto walls whilst carefully edging my way out of school, I made it home and stayed there. I became housebound, only able to go outside in a wheelchair.

Eating a more natural, primal-esque diet…

As part of my quest for health, I began to focus on natural, unprocessed, good quality foods; higher in protein and good fats. Eating a more caveman/ primal based diet I lowered my consumption of grains and sugar, instead acquiring carbohydrates mainly from vegetables and fruit. Without hesitation I adapted to my new primal-esque lifestyle, starting to eat unprocessed, natural foods in

9

the place of my old grain and sugar-based diet.

Within the next few months I was able to get up and walk around the house. I could do the small things which seem so trivial now such as standing up in the shower, making breakfast or even staying awake for longer than a couple of hours during the day. Ever so slowly I started to feel I could do more. I was less bloated, my abdominal pains faded away, my skin became smoother and healthier, colour returned to my face and my eyes had life back in them.

After a while having chicken and broccoli (however much I do actually love them) every day became a little monotonous, so during the times I was well enough to get up and about around the house, I became determined to make the most of my new way of eating. Excited about how my health was improving, I was adamant I would make the most out of the foods I could eat. There's no rule saying cakes have to be heavily processed, high in carbohydrates made with buckets of flour and heaps of refined sugars. So why couldn't I make a cake that I could eat? I'd just have to be a little creative...

So I spent the time I could in the kitchen trying to recreate the foods I had loved when I was younger and fashion them in a way that eliminated the grains and processed foods and incorporated the healthy wholesome foods I could eat.

In between recovering and studying at home, and then later at part time school for my A levels, I experimented. I noted down foods I fancied, combinations I thought would go together and how it could work. With my mum and sisters also being unwell it was incredibly important to me to be able to give the people that I loved, food that was good for them and mostly food they could enjoy again.

Once I reached a stage of health where I was able to get out and about by myself again, it became blindingly obvious that there weren't any fun healthy foods available. There were the heavily processed 'diet foods' and others, containing heaps of chemicals. However, after my health experiences I wanted to eat something tasty whilst still adhering to a healthier, more natural, lower carbohydrate lifestyle.

After a few frustrating trips out, wanting to know what was in my food when eating out, I decided to do something about it. That's what this book is all about, exploring food outside the usual grains and sugar-based diet, providing other options so people can still enjoy their favourite dishes but with a healthy twist. The influence and experience on this treatment and lifestyle encouraged me to write this book and start, 'Emily Jane's Foods®,' to offer real foodies, real food.

10

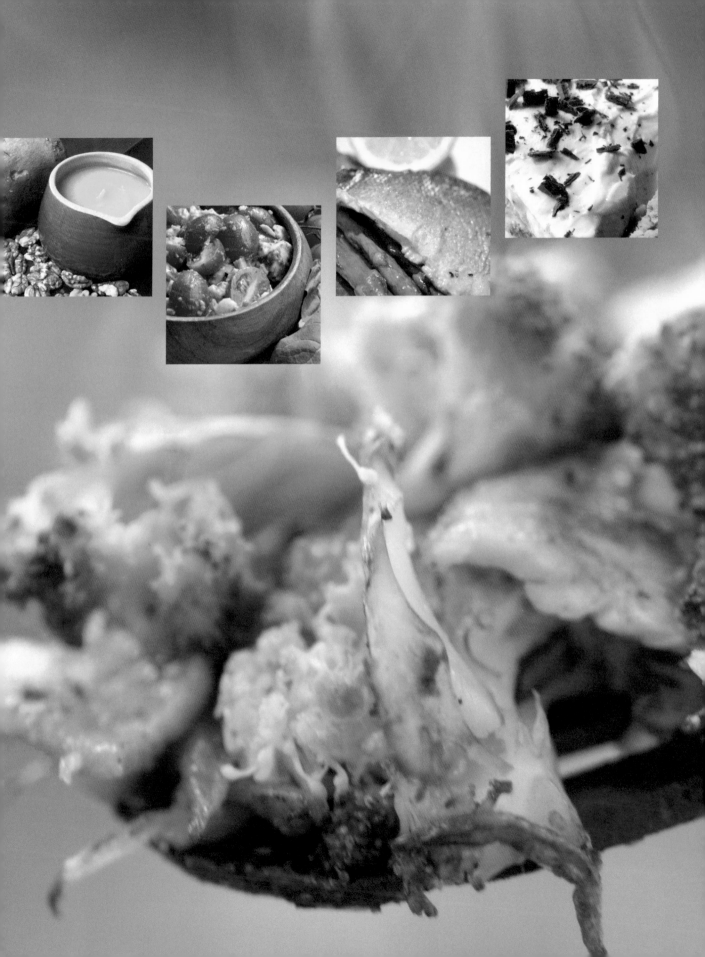

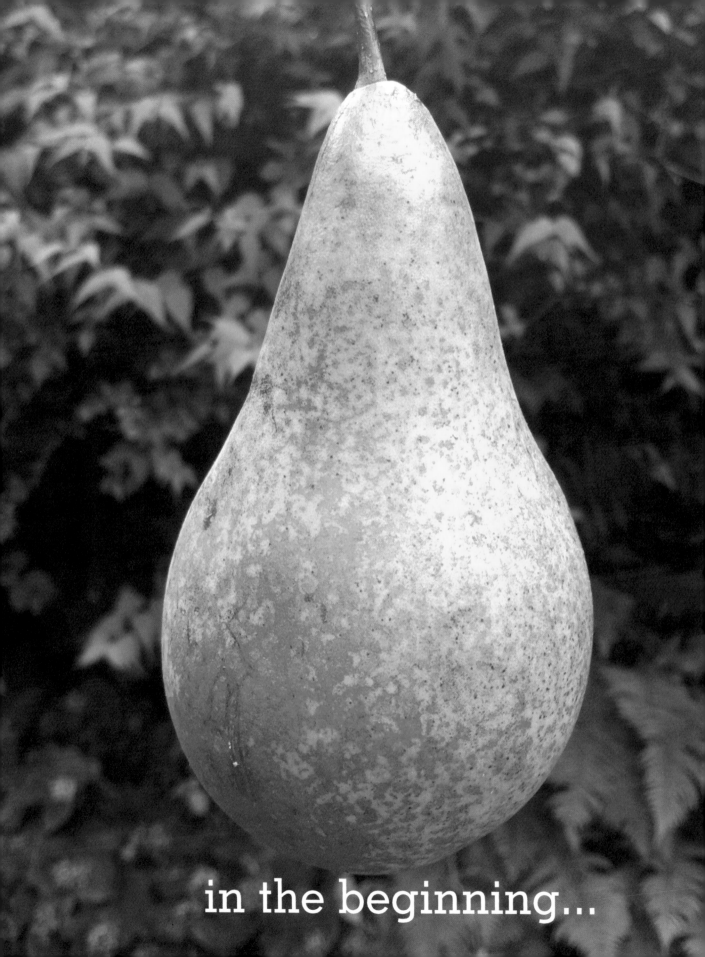

in the beginning...

..there was simple, fresh, natural food

Living off the land, eating good food; meat, veg, nuts, fruits, feeling satisfied on smaller amounts of nutritious meals. Slowly, over time, as the need to preserve food grew, we started to think up ways of making our food last longer. Additives and stabilisers were pumped in, to stop our food decaying as quickly. Finding grains were relatively cheap and easy to process, they were incorporated into everything. Practically no food remained untouched by grains and sugar.

Going from a place of simple, unadulterated nutrition, to large volumes of ingredients, processed and modified, we were hooked and carbohydrate cravings took hold. Weight gain became increasingly prevalent, dress sizes on the shelves exploded. Before long, everyone knew someone with crohns, insulin resistance or IBS. Diabetes and obesity became everyday words.

Being naturally inquisitive creatures, we began questioning what had caused this dramatic increase in ill health and disease. Blame had to lie somewhere. People started realising they gained weight when they ate cake or biscuits. Suddenly that pizza wasn't so healthy either, and in the midst of confusion, the finger of blame came to rest solely on fats. The cake and biscuits were stripped of butter, the pizza was topped with less cheese, pasta dishes had fewer or no toppings. Along with the loss of fat came a loss of flavour, taste and most importantly, satiety... the low fat trend had begun.

Hurrah everyone thought! That's the end of that. Soon supermarket shelves were filled with low fat (sneakily high sugar) options in a desperate attempt to decrease that number on the scales. But, for some reason, the weight gain didn't stop in its tracks and dwindle back down, instead, increasing further. Disease was on the increase.

Mixed messages and diet advice were thrown from every direction and confusion took hold. Nobody knew whether they should eat low fat, high protein, low carbohydrate, low protein, high fat, the next fashionable fad diet, etc...

Our food history doesn't make for such a wonderful story after all that.

I'm fascinated by food...

… different textures and tastes, the appearance. I find sitting down to eat a beautiful meal so much more satisfying than filling up on junk food or microwave meals. It's also an excuse to sit down and talk. Using the opportunity of a gorgeous meal as a social event, whether it's as big as a meal with friends or as small and cosy as a dinner for two. But ill health can cause food to lose its spark and trying to rectify the problem can sometimes be confusing, especially with mixed messages hitting from every angle. One minute we should be eating more fibre, then less fibre, then more protein will help you lose weight, but too much protein and your kidneys are in grave peril. Eat lots of

13

fruit and vegetables to get your vitamins and minerals, but you need to take multivitamins anyway and fruit contains a lot of fructose and that poisons the liver. Oh really? Meat is going to kill us all? Ok then, I'll get my protein from nuts and seeds but no wait, they contain fats and we can't have that. Eggs, perfect, I'll have an omelette... but what's this? There's a lot of cholesterol in egg yolks? Ok...

There are so many articles advocating certain health benefits and describing what we should and should not eat, but going completely back to basics, starting afresh, looking at what makes sense and what causes all the health problems that lead us to diet is the first step.

Here are the basics that I've found make sense to me;

Food is so abundant...

... that we eat whenever we want with little effort to obtain it. There are obvious positive implications with food being so easily accessible; not having to run after our dinner, with the prospect of going without and starving. Also supermarkets and the like can be a helpful, convenient option for certain ingredients. For example, tinned fresh fruits can be helpful to have on hand, as a matter of convenience, for those times when there aren't enough hours in the day, these can be a time saver and are much more beneficial than, say, a doughnut.

However, there are also negative implications. As minimal energy is needed to acquire our meals, we find ourselves in a position of

14

being able to eat as much and as often as we possibly can (funds allowing!), causing portion control to become a thing of the past. This creates a bit of a problem: many of us not knowing when to limit our food intake; with all we could want at our disposal, we don't even have to walk to our food source, so the exercise element is entirely eliminated.

It's not only the sheer volume of food that we ingest that has changed, but also nutrition type and quality. With the ever increasing population, the demand for food is higher than ever. It's no wonder cheaper foods and methods of production, in astoundingly large volumes, are appealing. Unfortunately this often compromises on food quality, usually involving large amounts of highly refined chemical fillers to make fewer ingredients stretch further, in order to feed more people as cheaply as possible.

Grains tend to form the base of our diets...

... and being a relatively new food source, our bodies are not designed to cope with consuming them, especially not in the vast quantities we are used to nowadays. For some people, intolerances to grains are not evident and they continue to eat them without obvious problems. However for a large proportion of us, heaps of grains prove to be much more trouble than they're worth - feeding harmful bacteria, exacerbating inflammation and disease processes, leading to intolerances and allergies.

Grains create problems for various reasons. Wheat in particular has become one of the better known allergies due to its infamous component; gluten. Gluten is the protein component in wheat which may encourage an inflammatory reaction in the body, causing trouble most commonly (but not exclusively) in the GI tract. Problems such as IBS, colitis and Crohns disease being the more commonly recognised.

Why is this a problem?

Harmful bacteria present in the body produce toxins, which, in turn, produce inflammation in the body and have been suggested to be the cause of many well-known diseases, such as the 'auto-immune' diseases; Poly-cystic ovarian syndrome (PCOS), obesity, autism, heart disease, the list goes on and on... These bacteria, using glucose as a fuel source to thrive and replicate are provided with an abundance of fuel with the high level of carbohydrates provided when grains and high levels of sugars and starches are consumed.

As humans, our bodies can only use carbohydrates in their simplest form, called monosaccharides. Common carbohydrate monosaccharides are glucose, fructose and lactose. When these monosaccharides are ingested, we can absorb them. When we eat starches, these are disaccharides (two monosaccharides joined together) or polysaccharides (chains of monosaccharides joined together); we must first break them down into monosaccharides before we can absorb them into the body. However, with the vast amount of starch consumed, large portions find themselves undigested in our intestines.

Some of this makes up the waste matter we build up in our bowels. However, also naturally present in our GI tract are a plethora of bacteria. These bacteria couldn't be happier, using these starches as a fuel source. As the harmful bacteria feed, they produce gas and acids. The gas given off gives us terribly unpleasant symptoms such as; flatulence, a general abdominal full feeling and bloating. The acids produced by harmful bacteria can also negatively affect the intestinal lining, destroying villi, which are involved in nutrient absorption in the intestines. This causes fewer nutrients from the food eaten, to be absorbed by the body and more nutrients to be used as a food source for the present harmful bacteria.

So theoretically you would think that monosaccharides (simple sugars eg glucose) are fine to eat on the premise that we can eat the foods which we can easily digest. However, this also appears to be a problem. Consuming large volumes of these monosaccharides in the form of glucose, fructose and lactose, not only fuels our cells and bodies but is also used as a food source for harmful bacteria and fungus (such as candida) throughout our bodies. These pathogens then also continue to multiply, becoming stronger than the individual's immune system, eventually overpowering the body's defences and causing a whole host of diseases. Some of these have been given the name 'auto-immune' or chronic inflammatory diseases. There has been conflict and confusion concerning the cause of these diseases but more research has begun to point towards bacteria playing a major role in the cause of these horrendously underplayed diseases.

Over the last few years, more attention has been directed to the problems of eating a diet containing a large amount of monosaccharides (sugar), in terms of obesity, the effects that the sugars have on the metabolism itself and the effect that they have on bacteria within the body.

One of the most infamous examples of the way a sugar-rich diet affects the body's metabolism, is the case of **insulin resistance and in some instances, the progression to diabetes**...

We have become accustomed to hearing that the hormone insulin plays a major role in regulating the metabolism of carbohydrates, transporting the glucose into cells for immediate use and storing any excess glucose as fats. Insulin has received a bad name, being known for creating fat stores. Yet surviving without this hormone would be impossible, as too much glucose in the bloodstream is 'toxic' (leading to severe metabolic disturbance and in extreme cases, coma), so insulin is required to round up circulating glucose in the bloodstream and package it into cells for storage. Being unable to properly detect and react to insulin heralds the first signs of insulin resistance. If this metabolic syndrome continues, the body needs more and more insulin to have the same effect until the pancreas cannot produce sufficient insulin to package the entirety of the carbohydrates consumed and diabetes starts.

GI (glycemic index)...

... is a scale used to measure the increase in insulin levels after eating a food. The specific food is appointed a GI number to indicate the increase of the insulin rise. The quicker and more steep the insulin release, the higher the GI value; the slower and the less steep the insulin release, the lower the GI value. Constant, sharp increases in insulin production are induced by consuming high sugar foods. Eating a lower GI diet aims to prevent these sharp insulin peaks.

Calories...

... have been subject to much scrutiny and the whole calories in vs calories out theory has been placed under the magnifying glass. As I see it, your body has to fulfil certain basic requirements to stay alive, and then additional requirements dependant on your energy output. Hence calories are needed for your BMR (Basal Metabolic Rate), daily movement, exercise. Any calories up until that point are used to fuel those actions, yet consuming further calories will cause the excess food to be stored in cells as fat.

This is a problem when consuming a diet rich in carbohydrates, as insulin levels are generally very high and the body is in a constant state of glucose burning. In other words the body is running on sugar. The residual fat stores created by the excess glucose being packaged into cells, would normally be broken down and released for use by glucagon. However, insulin and glucagon are antagonistic and so whilst high carbohydrate consumption and constant eating are maintained, insulin levels remain high and therefore the production of glucagon is suppressed. This means more sugar is stored as fat and the body is unable to burn off the fat stores without glucagon being present. Changing the food mix to a lower carbohydrate intake and to an increased protein and moderate fat consumption causes a decrease in insulin production. Glucagon is no longer inhibited and can therefore breakdown dietary fats and fat stores to be used by the body.

Prevention is better than cure.

Consuming fewer carbohydrates in the form of sugars and starches means providing less

ready nutrition for the bacteria living in our bodies, which may do us harm in the future. So before we find ourselves being handed lists of prescriptions and endless diagnoses, we can choose to help prevent this from happening. For those of us unfortunate enough to already have certain diseases, be it depression, IBS, Lyme disease or ME, wanting to get back to a level of good health is a focus. Getting rid of highly processed grains and immunosuppressive refined sugars, seems not only to discourage the disease from progressing, but also to give ourselves the best chance of recovery and hopefully give our immune systems a helping hand to fight the disease.

17

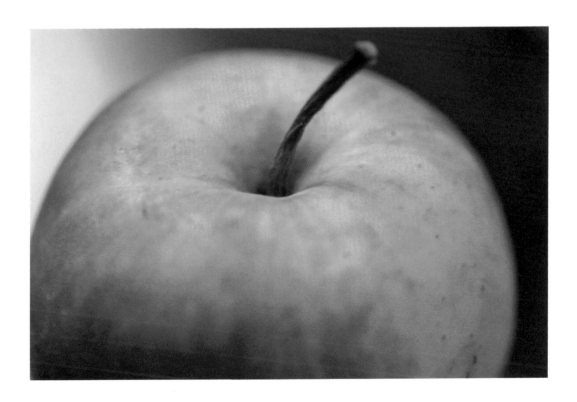

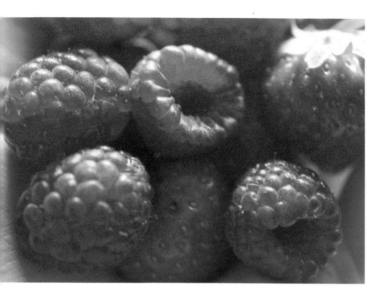

ingredients...

When writing this book, I wanted to include recipes which were suitable for everyone so as not to leave anyone out, whether you have a dairy intolerance, nut intolerance, or lead a vegetarian or vegan lifestyle. I soon realised that if I catered for absolutely everyone's requirements I wouldn't have many recipes at all. Either that or I'd have to write each recipe out several times with different substitutions or amendments. So instead, the recipes are written how I use them and what I think works best with the flavours of each individual dish. There is an array of dishes suitable for all kinds of diets and individual requirements. However for those of you who find the recipe you're looking for but find that there's a slight tweak needed with one of the ingredients, I've included some substitution suggestions below. The results may vary depending on the food substituted and certain recipes won't work with a substitution, for instance whipping a cream substitute to make whipped cream. I have written the most popular ones I can think of and will give some tips on the recipes themselves but the possibilities are endless so feel free to experiment!

Meat, Fish, Vegetables and Fruit

For any fresh produce I try to use good quality ingredients and organic wherever possible. It's important to get the best quality fresh produce possible as highly processed and some non-organic products can be devastating to your health. Meats which have been factory farmed have more often than not been pumped full of antibiotics and unnaturally high doses of vitamins and minerals which then get passed on to you through the food.

Mass-produced vegetables and fruits are often sprayed with dangerous chemicals and pesticides to keep pests at bay. However, many of these also remain intact when they reach us, meaning once again we ingest unnatural, harmful chemicals on otherwise healthy foods.

I'd rather get a better quality product than think of all that on my dinner plate... yuck.

Eggs

When flicking through this book you may notice that medium sized egg whites are predominantly used in the recipes. During my recovery, it was recommended that egg yolk consumption should be temporarily limited; hence most of my recipes exclude the egg yolk.

The baked goods are fairly inflexible and an egg yolk may have to be substituted into the recipe as simply adding it in will change the chemistry of the ingredients. However, for the more savoury dishes, for example the omelette pizza, the extra egg yolks will

...aargh, I can't have that!

change the flavour but can easily be added to the dish without too much change to the end product.

You can buy already separated egg whites to prevent wasting the yolks or use whole eggs and separate the white from the yolk. These spare egg yolks can then either be used in other dishes or if there isn't an immediate use for them, you could refrigerate or freeze them. Failing that, chuck a couple of the extra yolks into a breakfast omelette.

Nuts

Nuts are used a fair amount throughout this book. Nuts and nut butters are a nutrient-dense food, naturally high in good fats and protein and low in carbohydrates. As such they are high in calories and so should be eaten in moderation. Unlike using conventional wheat flour, each nut has its own distinctive taste, making them a perfect contribution to making each great tasting dish unique.

In particular, almonds are becoming increasingly available and are a popular

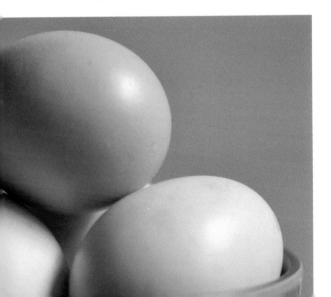

substitute for flour products. However when it comes to baked goods, ground almonds cannot be substituted as a 1:1 ratio for conventional grain flours. Ground almonds are less absorbent and due to the absence of gluten, it does not bond well, without a gelatinous effect forming. In which case, eggs can be used to bind the mixture, ensuring the foods don't crumble apart after one bite.

Chocolate

When I'm craving something gooey and sinfully chocolaty, I often prefer to use cocoa powder in my baking than chocolate. This way I can control what I use as a sweetener and exactly how sweet I want to make it.

There are times when a recipe calls for the chocolate to set, so in these cases I use a bar of good quality dark chocolate. When I do use bars of chocolate, as with all my sweeter foods, I use the smallest amounts possible and go for the highest cocoa percentage I can find, whilst still giving a deep chocolaty taste without being too bitter; this is usually about 70% cocoa content.

Sweetening

For all the sweeteners, I use the smallest amounts possible. When I started out creating different foods, I began experimenting with the artificial sweeteners range. However, every time I would trial an artificial sweetener I would read a disastrous account of potential negative health effects.

I decided it wasn't worth the risk. My health was already severely impaired and unwilling to further stack the odds against myself, I turned to more natural ingredients.

However, the amount of starch and sugar typically found in most commercial products was ridiculously excessive, meaning I had to experiment with other ingredients; starting from nothing and slowly tasting as I cooked, I managed to reach the desired level of sweetness without going overboard.

I soon discovered that such a large volume of sweet ingredients weren't necessary. I started to make large cakes with a tablespoon or two of honey and they turned out perfectly, pleasantly sweet.

The most common foods I use as sweeteners are honey, dates, fruits and dried fruits. There is no getting round it; these foods are high GI, but the way they are used in my recipes make the difference. The volume of these sweeter foods is as small as possible and as there are no flour/grain based ingredients, this means there is a decreased volume of starches present.

Butter, Oils and other fats

Fats such as butter, coconut butter, oils, coconut oil, seed butters and nut butters are great sources of protein and good fats, although these are high in calories, so if weight loss is on your agenda then eat these in moderation.

When substituting, each of the fats have different properties. Coconut butter and oils substitute well for butter but will change the flavour. Using seed butters or nut butters will add bulk to the product, making the product firmer and give the product a more individual taste.

Throughout this book, different fats are used for different recipes. In one I might use traditional butter, such as my Victoria sponge cake, whereas in others, I use olive oil, hazelnut oil, walnut oil, coconut oil or coconut butter. I have written each individual recipe with the types of fat that I feel fit the taste of that food especially well. Each one has different properties and different flavours to contribute to the overall taste and however appealing it would be to use just one fat source for all the recipes, I don't do this because I like the diversity of flavours and nutrients obtained from the different fats.

A bonus of doing this is that some of you reading this book may have a preference to one of the ingredients that I may not have used, had I stuck with using just one. Or others may have an intolerance to a certain ingredient. Usually substituting between the solid butters can be swapped at a 1:1 ratio. However, if swapping between a solid fat and liquid oil, a better substitution is 50g butter to 40ml oil.

Dairy

Crème fraiche and cream cheese make frequent appearances in bread rolls, pizza bases etc. The type you use is completely your choice. I tend to use half fat variations with no other additives, sugars or stabilisers added. If you're lactose intolerant, some of the dairy products such as milk and cream can be replaced by nut milks or creams.

20

equipment

Dried fruits

When using dried fruits as a source of sweetness as a topping or addition to a meal I try to always buy dried fruit without any added sugar or other additives. Try to avoid the dried fruits glazed in sugars or glucose syrups or tossed in flours to stop the pieces sticking together.

Oven

Throughout this book I use a fan-assisted oven. If you are going to use a regular oven then raise the temperature by approximately 10-20 degrees celcius or follow your oven manufacturer's instructions.

Processes

During baking I use a few processes which are different from those used in conventional baking.

Whipped egg whites – I frequently whisk the egg whites, usually to stiff peaks for use in baked goods. This helps give baked goods height and volume. When mixing in whipped egg whites, always fold them in gently, mixing in a crisscross pattern into the mixture until mixed in.

Dates – sometimes dates can be hard to use and if you find yourself without a high speed blender it can be difficult to break these down. In these cases I add the dates to a small saucepan with a small splash of water and heat on a low heat until the dates have absorbed the water, are softer and are able to be pureed or used in the recipe according to the recipes instructions.

Throughout this book different processes and certain equipment may be required to give the desired finish to the dish. I've compiled a brief list of equipment that is useful to have on hand:

- Hand blender
- Grater
- Hand held julienne slicer – one of the best buys ever
- High-speed blender or hand blender
- Large and small saucepans
- Frying pan
- Oven with a fan assisted and grill setting
- Waffle maker
- Sieve
- Large mixing bowls
- Electric whisk
- Nut and seed grinder

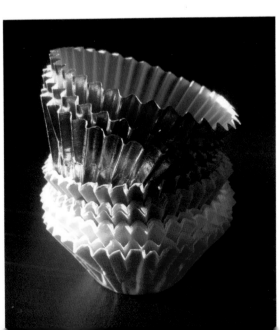

BREAD AND MILK ARE TWO OF THE MOST
POPULAR STAPLES. FORMING THE BASE OF
MOST OF OUR DIETS, WE CAN'T BEAR TO
THINK OF LIFE WITHOUT OUR TOAST AND
CEREAL WITH MILK IN THE MORNING, SOFT
FILLED ROLLS AND WRAPS AT LUNCH AND A
CREAMY HOT CHOCOLATE TO SEND US OFF
TO BED. FOR THOSE WITH INTOLERANCES
OR LOOKING FOR AN ALTERNATIVE TO THE
USUAL DAIRY MILK AND STARCHY BREADS,
THESE GIVE BACK OPTIONS FOR THE MORE
SIMPLE CONVENIENT FOODS AND CAN BE
USED FOR CERTAIN RECIPES THROUGHOUT
THIS BOOK

beautiful basics

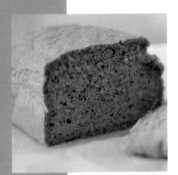

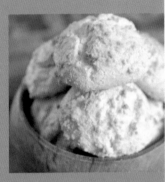

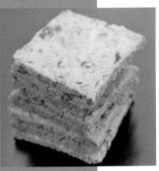

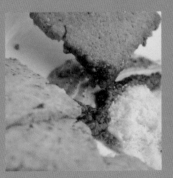

For most people, considering life without bread is unthinkable. Toast for breakfast, lunchtime sandwiches, bread basket starters at restaurants. Giving up a food so convenient and such an everyday base for most meals is difficult. So armed with this bread recipe you'll be well equipped for those times when only a bacon sarni will do.

24

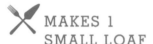 MAKES 1
SMALL LOAF

100g cashew butter

4 egg whites

Large pinch sea salt

1 tablespoon lemon juice

½ teaspoon bicarbonate soda

White bread

- Preheat the oven to 160 degrees (fan assisted oven)

- Blend together the cashew butter, one egg white, salt, lemon juice and bicarbonate soda

- Whisk the remaining 3 egg whites until they reach stiff peaks

- Add the egg whites, a third at a time, to the cashew butter mixture and cut into the mixture to mix together, without knocking the air out of the batter

- Pour the batter into a lined 1lb bread tin and place in the oven for 30-40 minutes or until the top is turning brown and firm to the touch

- Once cooked, remove from the oven and leave to cool

- Once cooled, slice and use immediately or wrap in cling film and store in the fridge

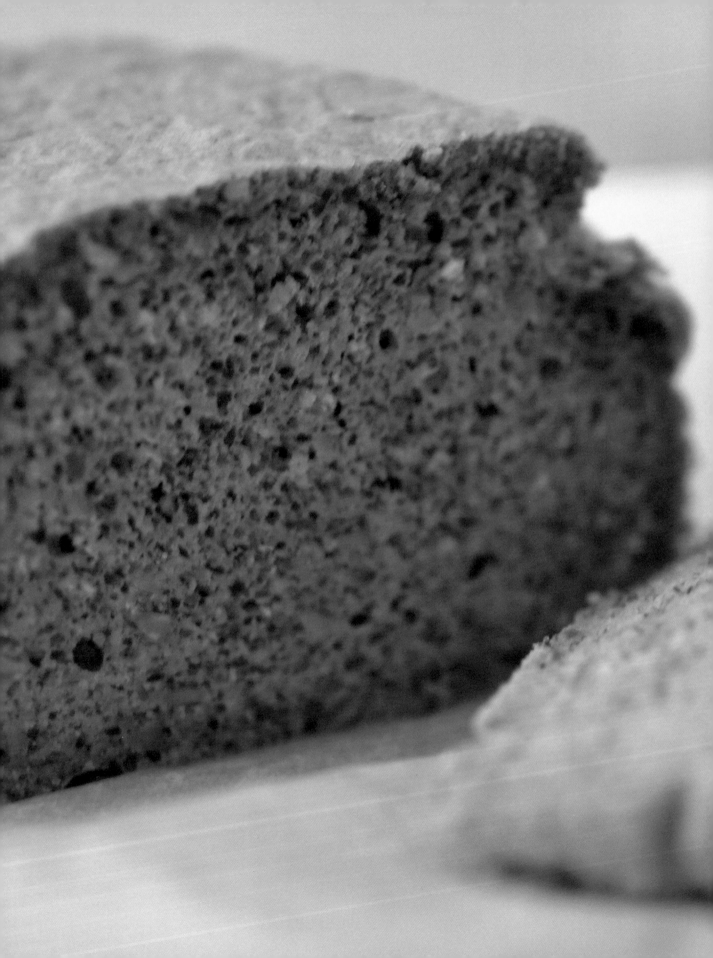

❝ The seeds in this loaf provide extra crunch and texture to the slices ❞

Brown bread

- Preheat the oven to 160 degrees (fan assisted oven)

- Blend together the almond butter, one egg white, salt, lemon juice and bicarbonate soda

- Whisk the remaining 3 egg whites until they reach stiff peaks

- Add the egg whites, a third at a time, to the cashew butter mixture and cut into the mixture to mix together, without knocking the air out of the batter

- Pour the batter into a lined 1lb bread tin and place in the oven for 30-40 minutes or until the top is turning brown and firm to the touch

- Once cooked, remove from the oven and leave to cool

- Once cooled slice and use immediately or wrap in cling film and store in the fridge

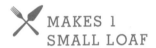 **MAKES 1 SMALL LOAF**

100g roasted almond butter

Handful pumpkin seeds

4 egg whites

½ teaspoon bicarbonate of soda

20ml water

1 teaspoon lemon juice

Large pinch of salt

27

Great with any filling, these can be made into small buns or longer rectangular shapes to make a Panini. Made into small buns, these are great little sandwiches. Drop the mixture into a longer oblong shape. Once cooked, cut in half lengthways and fill with pesto, mozzarella, ribbons of ham, sliced tomatoes, a small handful of cheese, any fillings you want. Then toast the Panini in a flat plated sandwich toaster for a few minutes, until slightly flattened and warmed through.

28

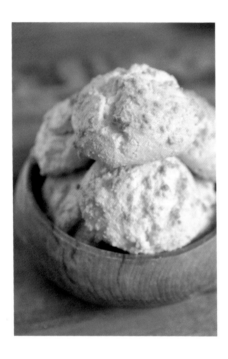

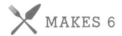 MAKES 6

2 egg whites

100g low fat cream cheese

1 teaspoon white wine vinegar

½ teaspoon bicarbonate soda

150g ground almonds

Pinch coarse sea salt

Bread rolls

- Preheat the oven on 170 degrees celsius (fan assisted oven)

- In a first bowl whisk the egg whites until it forms stiff peaks

- In a second bowl mix together the cream cheese and white wine vinegar

- Add to this, the ground almonds, salt and bicarbonate soda and mix in

- Add a quarter of the egg whites at a time to the mixture, folding in the egg whites gently

- Once the mixture is incorporated, drop the mixture onto the greaseproof paper in neat, circular balls

- Bake in the oven for approx 20 minutes or until turning slightly brown and cooked through

- Remove from the oven and leave to cool before slicing and filling

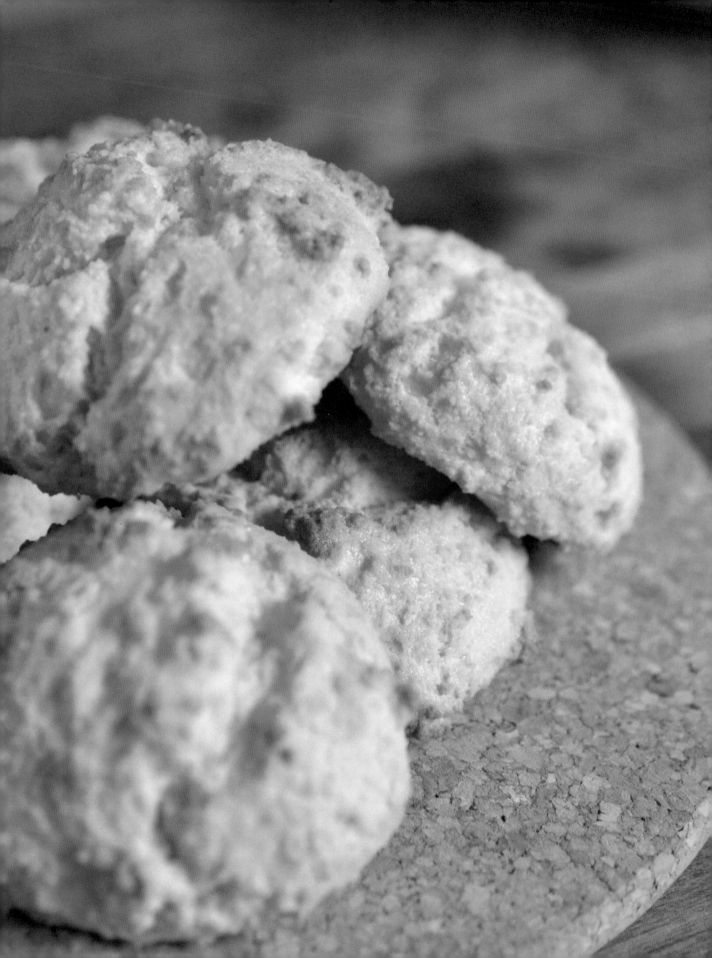

‘I reserve making loaves of bread for the occasional sandwich or my favourite bread related use – eggy bread. However, when I'm looking for a lighter lunch I make a quick wrap coupled with my favourite fillings. Sweet or savoury, the options are endless...’

Wraps

✕ MAKES ONE WRAP

1 egg white

2 tablespoons ground almonds

1 tablespoon water

Pinch salt

- With a hand blender, blend together all the egg white, ground almonds, salt and water until smooth
- Heat a splash of olive oil in a non-stick frying pan on low to medium heat
- Pour the mixture into the pan and swirl the mixture to cover the base of the pan
- Once the first side is cooked and turning brown, very gently flip it over and cook on the other side until the wrap is firm and slightly brown on both sides
- Remove from the heat and leave on a plate to cool
- Once cooled, add your fillings and roll up the wrap

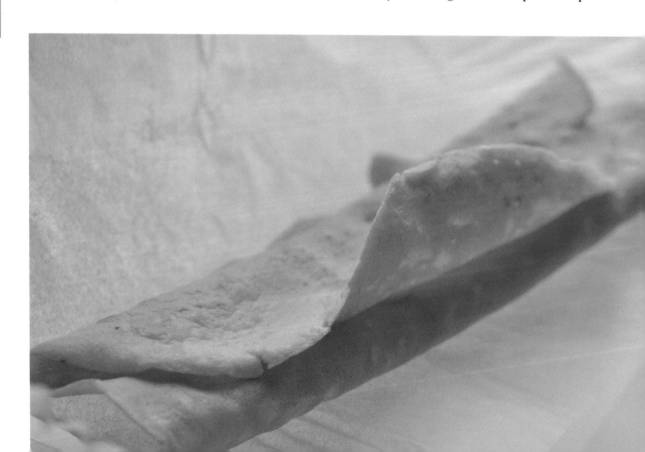

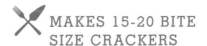

Perfect crackers for dips or try topped with a slice of cheese... mmm...

Salty walnut and oregano crackers

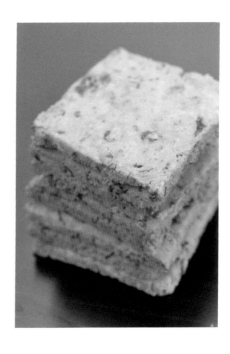

MAKES 15-20 BITE SIZE CRACKERS

1 egg white

¼ teaspoon coarse sea salt

½ teaspoon oregano

1 tablespoon olive oil

100g ground almonds

50g walnuts

- Preheat the oven to 160 degrees celsius (fan assisted oven)

- Add the egg white, salt, oregano and olive oil to a bowl and mix

- Add the ground almonds

- Chop the walnuts into small chunks and add these to the mixture

- Mix together until it forms a dough

- To roll out the dough, sandwich the dough between the two sheets of greaseproof paper

- Take a rolling pin and roll the dough until it's about ¼ inch tall

- Remove the top sheet of paper and cut the dough into squares, using a spatula to carefully move the squares onto a baking sheet

- Repeat this process until all the dough has been cut into squares

- Cook the squares in the oven for about 20 minutes or until turning golden brown

- Remove from the oven and leave to cool for 30 minutes

- Once cooled keep crackers in a sealable plastic bag or a glass jar with a sealable lid

31

Pesto with its beautifully salty taste was made to go with crackers. Here I decided to cut out the middle man, incorporating the pesto, making wonderfully salty, snappy crackers.

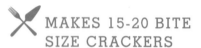

MAKES 15-20 BITE SIZE CRACKERS

2 tablespoons pesto

1 egg white

1 tablespoon coconut flour

100g ground almonds

1 heaped tablespoon parmesan (optional)

32

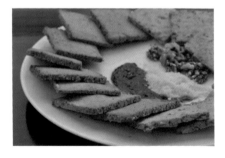

Pesto crackers

- Preheat the oven to 160 degrees celsius (fan assisted oven)

- Add the pesto, egg white and coconut flour to a bowl and mix

- Add the ground almonds and parmesan and mix together until it forms a dough

- To roll out the dough, sandwich the dough between the two sheets of greaseproof paper

- Take a rolling pin and roll the dough until it's about ¼ inch tall

- Remove the top sheet of paper and cut the dough into squares, using a spatula to carefully move the cut squares onto a baking sheet

- Repeat this process until all the dough has been cut into squares

- Cook the squares in the oven for about 20 minutes or until turning golden brown

- Remove from the oven and leave to cool for 30 minutes

- Once cooled keep crackers in a sealable plastic bag or a glass jar with a sealable lid

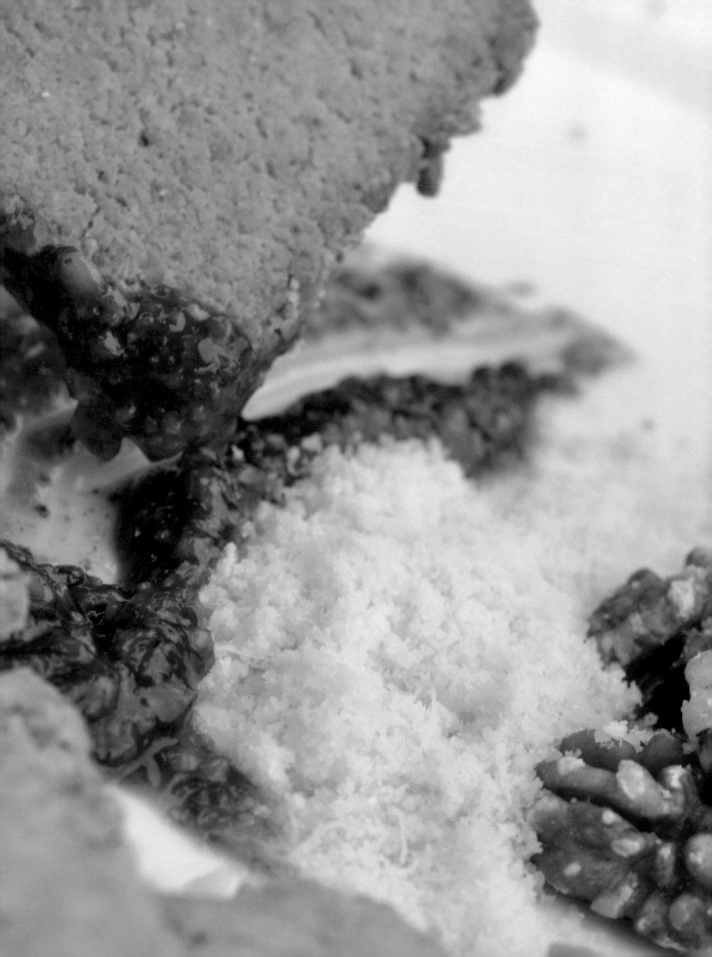

Coconut milk has been used in dishes for years, traditionally found in curries. Widely available in supermarkets and health stores alike. You can buy the canned coconut milk variety but I prefer using block coconut cream. Unlike most canned varieties, there are no stabilisers or additives, just 100% coconut flesh. Block coconut is also incredibly easy to use. You can make coconut milk and coconut cream, use it to thicken sauces, change the consistency by either adding more water or more coconut. Easy to use in a diverse range of dishes.

Coconut milk

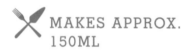 MAKES APPROX. 150ML

25g coconut block

150ml water

- Chop the coconut block into smaller pieces and add to a saucepan on low heat

- Once the coconut starts to melt, add the water to the saucepan

- Stir the mixture until all the coconut has melted and the liquid is consistently white

- Remove from the heat and leave to cool

- Once cool, pour the coconut milk into a flask and place in the fridge

- For coconut cream, continue to simmer the coconut milk, causing more of the water to evaporate off, until a thicker consistency is reached

Cashew milk is a gorgeous base in drinks, dairy free ice creams and as a dairy free milk or cream substitute. Cashew milk is more gentle on the stomach than fibrous coconut milk and gives a wonderfully naturally sweet, nutty taste. Like coconut milk, this is an easily flexible recipe and can be adjusted by adding more nuts or more water to change the consistency.

Sweet cashew milk

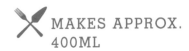 MAKES APPROX. 400ML

400ml water

50g cashew nuts (plain)

50g dates

Few drops vanilla essence

Pinch sea salt

35

- Chop the dates and add to a pan with a few tablespoons of the water and add to a saucepan to simmer on a low heat
- Grind the cashew nuts until they make a coarse flour
- Once the dates have softened, add the cashew pieces, the rest of the water, vanilla essence and salt
- Blend with a hand blender until you reach a smooth consistency
- Remove from the heat when the mixture reaches a milky consistency
- Leave to cool before placing in a covered container in the fridge
- If you would like a sweet pouring cream, keep simmering the mixture until it reaches a thicker creamy consistency

SOUPS ARE IDEAL AS A QUICK, WARM, COMFORTING SOURCE OF NUTRITION. HOWEVER, MOST SOUPS ON SUPERMARKET SHELVES OR AVAILABLE IN CAFES AND RESTAURANTS CONTAIN ADDITIVES, ALARMING AMOUNTS OF SUGAR FOR A SAVOURY DISH, ADDITIVES AND THICKENERS. CHOOSING TO EAT SOUP MADE FROM NATURAL, WHOLESOME INGREDIENTS ENABLES YOU TO KNOW WHAT IS GOING INTO YOUR BODY, SO YOU CAN CURL UP AND RELAX WITH YOUR BOWLFUL

silky smooth soups

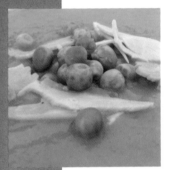

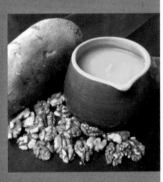

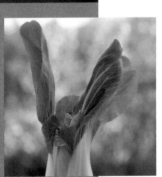

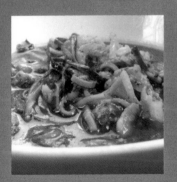

37

A nutritious staple most commonly used as a base for soups or gravy. Unlike most stock cubes containing highly processed oils and sugars, this stock gives off a fresh aromatic smell with a subtle flavour. You can always save juices from any roasts you make and add to the stock to increase the flavour. Here I use chicken legs with the meat still intact, using the leftover meat for stir-fries or adding to salads.

Essential chicken stock

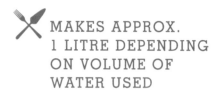 MAKES APPROX. 1 LITRE DEPENDING ON VOLUME OF WATER USED

4 chicken legs or one whole chicken carcass

2 carrots

1 leek

1 onion

2 sticks celery

Sea salt to taste

Large pinch white pepper

1 bouquet garni

2 bay leaves

Enough water to cover

- Roughly chop the carrots, leek and celery

- Add the chicken, chopped vegetables and white pepper, bay leaves and bouquet garni to a saucepan and cover with water

- Bring to the boil for 3 minutes then cover and reduce to a very low heat, leaving it simmering for one to one and a half hours

- Finely chop the onion and in a separate frying pan, sauté the onion in olive oil on a low heat until soft and slightly golden round the edges

- Add the sautéed onion to the stock

- Remove the chicken once cooked through and strip the meat off the bone. You will know the chicken is cooked through when the meat practically falls off the bone

- Place the bones back in the pan

- Leave to simmer to reduce the stock, adding salt to taste

- Sieve the contents of the pan, separating the stock from the veg and bones (word of warning; be careful not to pour the stock away, catching the solid in the sieve and watching your stock disappear down the sink drain. I make this mistake far more often than I like to admit...)

- Use immediately or allow to cool and store in a sealed container in the fridge

38

Broccoli and pea soup

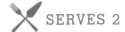 *Makes a light silky garden pea soup. Add ham for a wonderful pea and ham soup.*

- Finely chop the onion and in a saucepan, lightly sauté in olive oil until transparent
- Break up the broccoli into smaller florets and add to the pan along with the peas, followed by the chicken stock and salt.
- Bring to the boil
- After boiling for 2 minutes, lower temperature and leave to simmer for 10 minutes
- Once cooked use a blender to blend the mixture until there are no lumps
- Serve hot with a few chunks of fresh ham and peas to garnish

SERVES 2

1 large onion

2 tablespoons olive oil

½ head broccoli

300ml peas

Coarse sea salt

500ml chicken stock

39

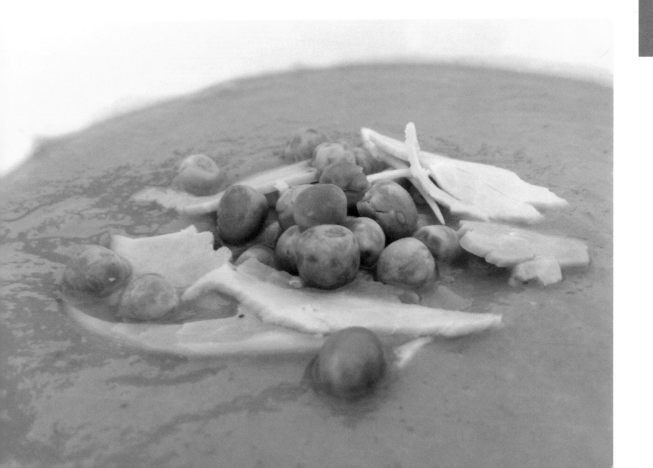

A vibrant soup with a subtle spicy kick.

Roasted pepper and tomato soup

SERVES 2

2 tablespoons olive oil

½ orange pepper

½ red pepper

250ml tomato passata

300ml chicken stock

3 tablespoons lentils

1 onion

1 teaspoon herbes de Provence

½ teaspoon smoked sea salt (normal coarse sea salt could alternatively be used)

½ teaspoon paprika

1/4 teaspoon white pepper

Black pepper to taste

40

- Finely chop the onions and sauté in olive oil with the chopped red pepper in a saucepan on a low heat

- Add the spices, salt, herbs and white pepper to the pan and stir occasionally

- Add the tomato passata, chicken stock and lentils

- Bring to the boil and place the lid on the saucepan for 10 minutes

- It's important to thoroughly cook the lentils, reduce the heat and simmer for approximately 30-40 minutes

- Once cooked through, pour the contents of the pan into a blender or use a hand blender to blend to a smooth consistency

- Serve whilst hot

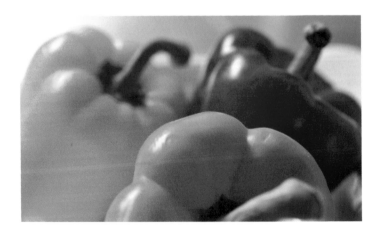

Thick watercress soup

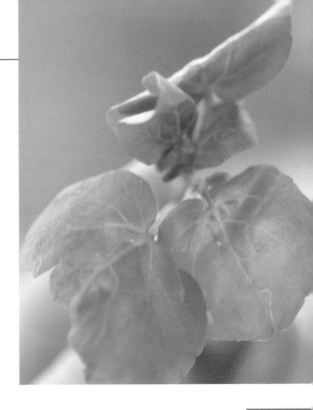

- Finely chop the onion and sauté in the olive oil on a low heat

- Add the salt and white pepper

- Roughly chop the cauliflower into smaller pieces and add to the pan to briefly sauté, giving the cauliflower some colour

- Add the chicken stock

- Bring to the boil for 2 minutes and then reduce the heat and leave to simmer for 10 minutes or until the cauliflower is cooked through

- Add the watercress at the last minute and remove from the heat

- Use a blender to blend the saucepan contents to produce a smooth, stomach warming soup

- Serve

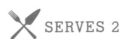 SERVES 2

41

1 onion

3 tablespoons olive oil

½ cauliflower head (approximately 250g)

¼ tsp coarse sea salt

⅛ tsp white pepper

500ml chicken stock

75g watercress

THE guilt free comfort soup, thick and fresh with a subtle peppery flavour. Viscous soups are often thickened with a traditional starchy thickener. However, this soup uses the cauliflower to give it a thick, smooth feeling for some guilt free comfort food.

If I had to award prizes to the most comforting vegetables (as one does), the sweet potato and butternut squash would definitely make the grade. Besides the attractive autumnal colours, they are also packed full of nutrients and flavour.

Sweet potato and butternut squash soup

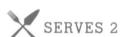 **SERVES 2**

1 large onion

2 tablespoons olive oil

¼ tsp coarse sea salt

⅛ tsp white pepper

150g sweet potato

150g butternut squash

350ml chicken stock

42

- Finely chop the onion

- Add to a saucepan on medium heat with the olive oil, salt, white pepper and sauté the onions until they start turning slightly brown

- Add the sweet potato and butternut squash and lightly fry for a minute or two

- Add the chicken stock and bring to the boil

- Leave the soup boiling for 2 or 3 minutes and then bring it back to medium heat and put the saucepan lid on

- After 10-15 minutes remove from the heat

- Use a blender to blend the contents of the saucepan until smooth and silky

- Serve

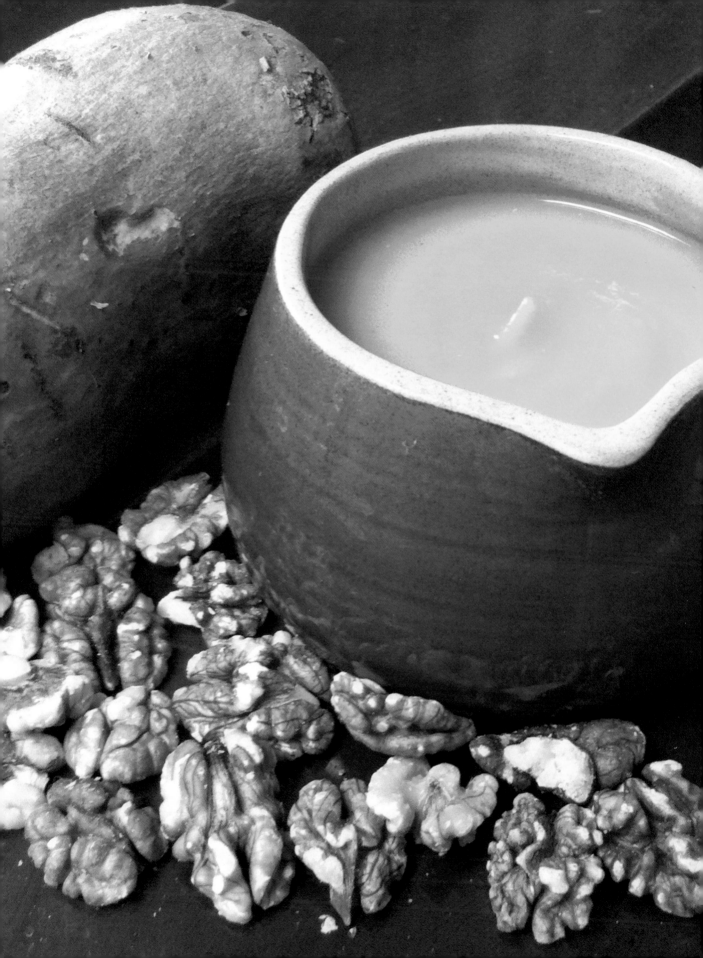

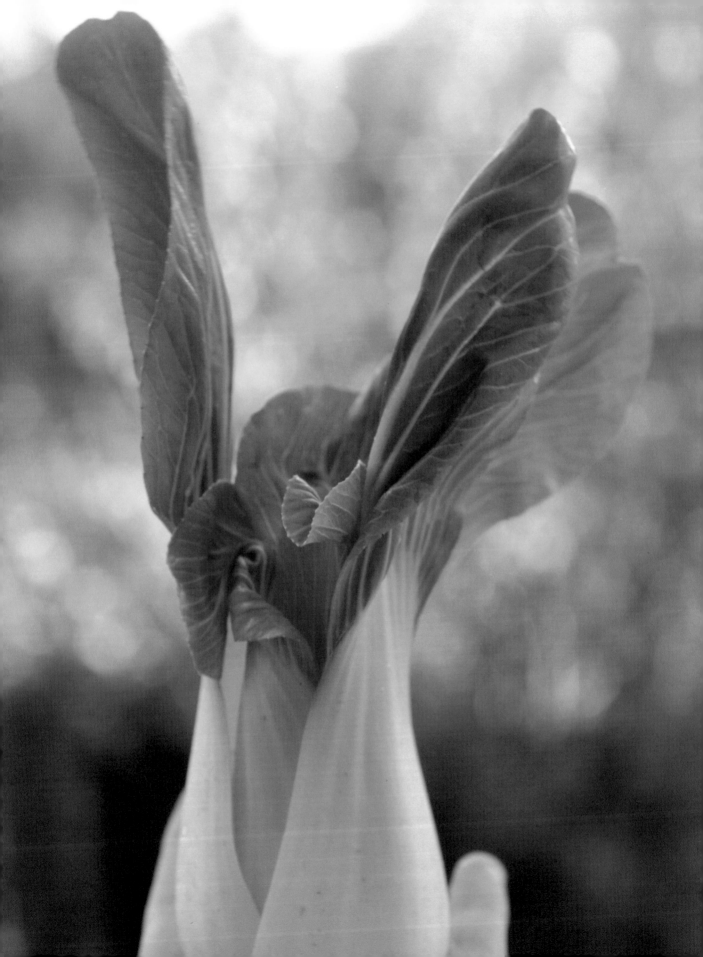

Mildly spicy, buttery textured soup, dotted with meatballs.

Pak choi with meatballs

Making the Meatballs:

- Add the sea salt and white pepper to the pork mince

- Mix all together thoroughly with your hands

- Then break off small amounts of mixture and roll into balls in your hands

- In a frying pan, brown the balls in the butter and olive oil on a medium heat

- Once browned, set aside and begin the soup

Soup:

- Finely chop the onion and sauté in the butter and olive oil

- Chop the leek and add to the pan

- Add the ginger, coriander, white pepper, cayenne pepper and salt

- Add the balsamic vinegar and water

- Chop the coconut block as finely as possible and add to the pan

- Wait till the coconut is almost completely melted and then add the water

- Add the meatballs to the soup and bring to the boil

- Cover and lower the heat and simmer for 15 minutes

- Add the Pak choi and simmer for a further few minutes

- Serve

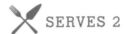 **SERVES 2**

1 onion

1 tablespoon butter

1 leek

¼ teaspoon ginger

¼ teaspoon coriander

Pinch white pepper

Pinch cayenne pepper

¼ teaspoon coarse sea salt

25g coconut cream block

1 tablespoon balsamic vinegar

800ml water

1 head pak choi

Meatballs:

500g pork mince

½ teaspoon coarse sea salt

⅛ teaspoon white pepper

Fry in a splash of olive oil

45

Pesto noodle soup

MAKES 1 LARGE BOWL

1 onion

1 tablespoon olive oil

1 tablespoon pesto

1 courgette

1 sausage

1 rasher of bacon

Small handful of leftover chicken

500ml chicken stock

- In a frying pan, cook the sausages and bacon

- Once cooked through, remove from the frying pan and set aside

- Finely chop the onion and sauté in the olive oil on a low heat until soft and turning golden brown

- Using a julienne slicer, slice the courgettes into long thin strips (otherwise cut courgettes into long thin strips) and add to the pan

- Once the courgette starts to turn soft and flexible, add the chicken stock and pesto

- Bring to the boil for 2 minutes and reduce to a simmer for 5 minutes

- Cut up the meat and add, continuing to simmer for a further 5 minutes

- Once the soup is heated through, serve

Absolutely packed with protein, I like to use good quality sausages and bacon in this soup, along with the chicken I usually have left over from my chicken stock.

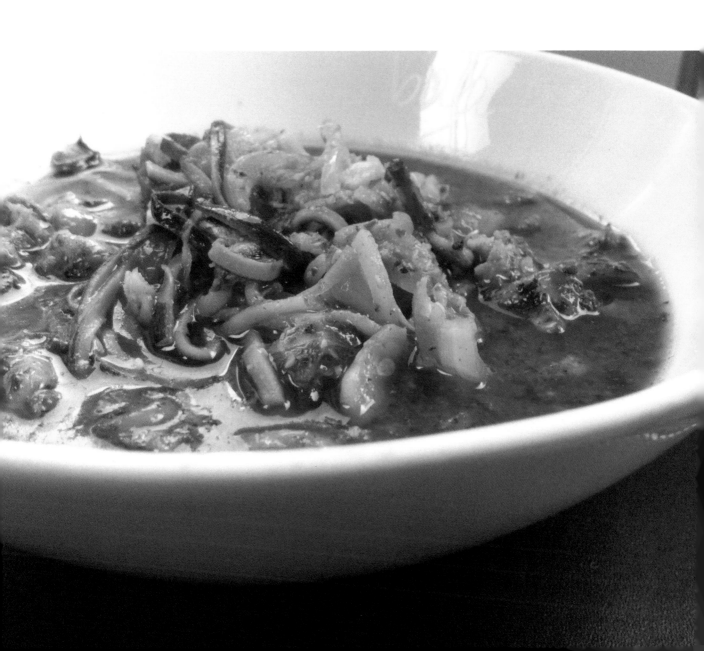

MAIN COURSES NOWADAYS TEND TO INVOLVE SERVINGS OF GARGANTUAN PORTIONS, WITH A LARGE PERCENTAGE OF THE MEAL BEING PILED HIGH WITH RICE, POTATOES, PASTA OR BREAD FOLLOWED BY A COMPARATIVELY MEAGRE SERVING OF MEAT AND VEGETABLES. INSTEAD, MAKING VEGETABLES THE MAIN BULK OF THE MEALS, OFTEN WITH A GENEROUS MEAT COMPONENT, DECREASES THE STARCHES AND PROVIDES A WHACKING DOSE OF PROTEIN AND NUTRIENTS. BUT THAT DOESN'T MEAN COMPROMISING ON TASTE. BY REMODELLING OLD FAVOURITES, WE CAN HAVE A POWERFULLY NUTRITIOUS MEAL ALONG WITH SIMPLE, BEAUTIFUL FLAVOURS

magnificent
meals

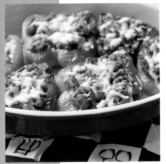

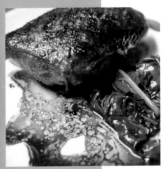

49

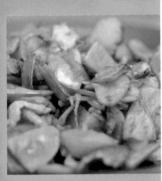

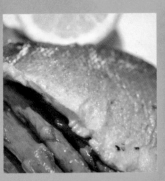

Aubergine, parmesan, tomato layers

✕ SERVES 4

3 aubergines

4 tablespoons olive oil

1 large onion

2 teaspoons basil

1 teaspoon oregano

¼ teaspoon coarse sea salt

⅛ teaspoon white pepper

600g chopped tomatoes

75g grated parmesan cheese

- Preheat the oven to 180 degrees celsius (fan assisted oven)

- Slice the aubergines into half a centimetre thick circles and place in a colander

- Salt the aubergine slices and leave to drain for an hour or so – aubergines can taste bitter if this step is missed out

- Whilst waiting for the aubergines to drain, finely chop the onion and fry with the olive oil in a saucepan on low heat

- Once turning translucent, add the basil, oregano, salt and white pepper

- Continue to cook until the onion turns golden brown

- Add the chopped tomatoes, stir and cook for about 10 minutes on low to medium heat and set aside

- Rinse the aubergine slices with water

- Heat a frying pan and fry the aubergine slices on both sides in a splash of olive oil

- Cover the bottom of a casserole dish with the grilled sliced aubergine, pour a third of the tomato sauce on top of this, then sprinkle a layer of parmesan on top

- Repeat this layering pattern until all the ingredients are used up

- Cook in the oven for approximately 40 minutes

- Once cooked, remove from the oven and serve whilst still warm

❝On Wednesday nights, my dad and I set aside an hour or two to go out for dinner. With our busy, separate lives it's a time reserved to catch up and have a chat about work or the week's events. Sometimes we'll just go for a drink and a quick chat but occasionally we'll have a meal out. On these occasions, a more frequent dinner choice has been a contemporary, low-key tapas restaurant in the town centre, where I found a new comfort dish to add to my favourites. This layered meal has all the rustic charm of a tagine dish, whilst giving the reminiscent layered look and taste of lasagne.❞

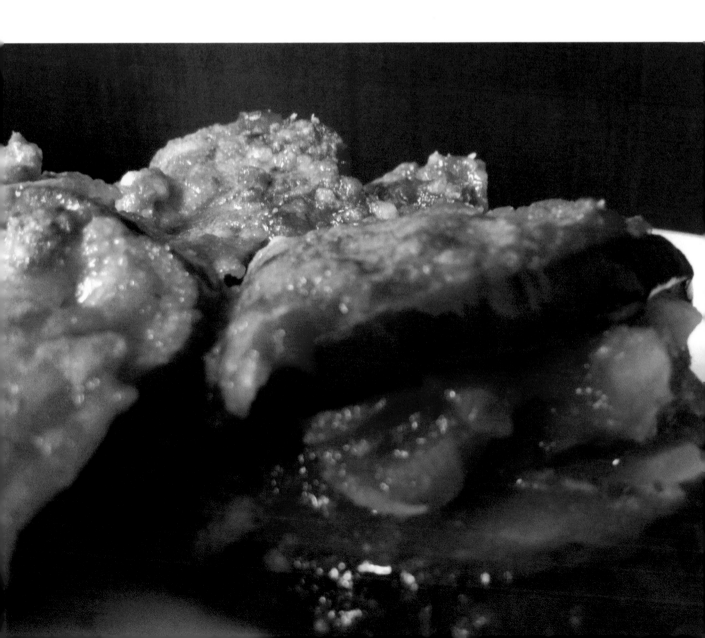

A big fan of chicken nuggets, these hit the spot when I get that fast food craving. With a pot of super quick homemade tomato ketchup on the side, it's a case of ready, steady, dunk...

Chicken nuggets

- In a bowl combine the ground almonds, salt, white pepper and cayenne pepper
- Place the chicken breasts between 2 pieces of cling film and tenderise (read; stress release) until approximately half a centimetre thick
- Heat up the walnut oil in a large frying pan on high heat
- Cut each flattened chicken breast into bite size pieces
- Then add the ground almonds and mustard to the bowl with the chicken
- Use your hands to completely coat the chicken in the mixture
- Toss the chicken strips in the pan
- Cook for approximately 5 minutes or until brown on the outside and cooked through, regularly turn the chicken bites over
- Serve with a large side of tomato ketchup and coleslaw

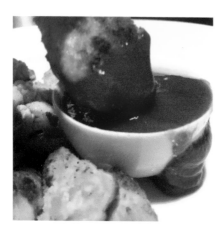

52

SERVES 4

4 chicken breasts

50g ground almonds

1 teaspoon coarse sea salt

Large pinch white pepper

½ teaspoon Dijon mustard

Large pinch cayenne pepper

Walnut oil

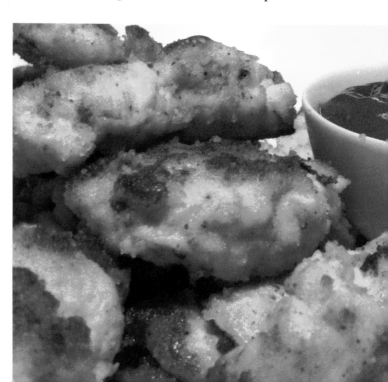

Creamy chicken satay

Creamy peanut butter satay sauce with chunks of mango, smothered over chicken pieces. Use a julienne slicer to cut super fine cucumber noodles as an accompaniment for this dish.

- Melt the coconut block in the saucepan with the water on a low heat

- Once the coconut has melted add the peanut butter, mild chilli powder, ginger, cumin and balsamic vinegar and stir

- Add salt to taste

- Tear up pieces of cooked chicken (I use leftover roasted chicken for this recipe but you could also chop up and stir fry some chicken thighs or breast and add this to the sauce)

- Chop the mango into small cubes and add to the saucepan

- As all the chicken is already cooked, the chicken satay only needs to be heated, so leave on a medium heat until hot then remove from the heat

- Using a julienne slicer, julienne the cucumber lengthways into long thin strips – if you don't have a julienne slicer to hand, slice the cucumber lengthways into very thin strips

- Place the cucumber noodles in a bowl and pour the satay over the top

- To finish the dish, finely chop a spring onion and sprinkle over the top

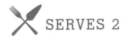 SERVES 2

¼ teaspoon mild chilli powder

¼ teaspoon ginger

⅛ teaspoon cumin

Coarse sea salt to taste

25g coconut

100ml water

4 tablespoons chunky peanut butter

1 teaspoon balsamic vinegar

2 roasted chicken legs (or other cooked chicken pieces)

½ mango

1 cucumber

1 spring onion

53

This dish oozes colour with the beautiful red, orange and yellow boats, stuffed with seasoned mince and salty chunks of bacon, these are a frequent visitor in the Whiteley household

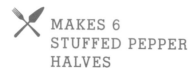 MAKES 6
STUFFED PEPPER
HALVES

3 peppers red, orange, yellow, or a combination to make it colourful, whichever you prefer

Olive oil

Sea salt

Filling:

500g pork mince

1 teaspoon coarse sea salt

1 teaspoon sage

¼ teaspoon ground mixed spice

Pinch white pepper

100g grated cheddar cheese

3 rashers bacon

Stuffed peppers

- Preheat the oven to 180 degrees celsius (fan assisted oven)

- Slice the peppers in half, removing the stalks and seeds from the inside

- After washing the peppers halves, pour a generous amount of olive oil and crush the salt, rubbing them on to the peppers and place in a casserole dish

- Roast in the oven for approx 40 minutes

- Whilst the peppers are roasting, fry the bacon rashers in a frying pan on medium heat until crispy, remove from the pan and set aside

- Add the sage, ground mix spice, white pepper and salt to the mince and, using your hands, incorporate the seasonings into the mince, mixing well

- Drain off most of the bacon juices left in the pan, leaving a little for frying a finely chopped onion on a low heat

- Add to this the pork mince and brown for about 10 minutes on medium heat

- Once the mince is browned, turn off the heat

- Chop the bacon rashers into small squares and add to the mince

- Also add 50g of the grated cheddar cheese and give the mince a quick stir to incorporate all the ingredients

- When the peppers are slightly crinkly on the surface and are much softer, remove from the oven

- Once cool enough to touch, spoon the mince mixture into each of the pepper halves, enough to adequately fill each to the top

- Once filled, sprinkle the remaining 50g grated cheese to top the stuffed peppers

- Place back in the oven for another 30-40 minutes, or until cooked through

- Once cooked, remove the tray from the oven and serve whilst still hot

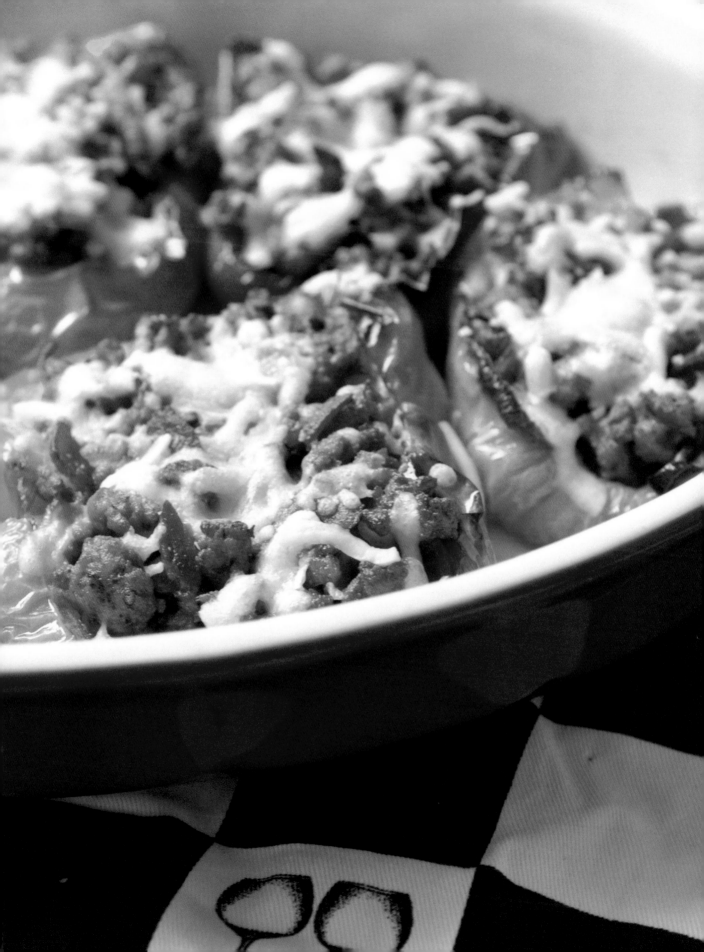

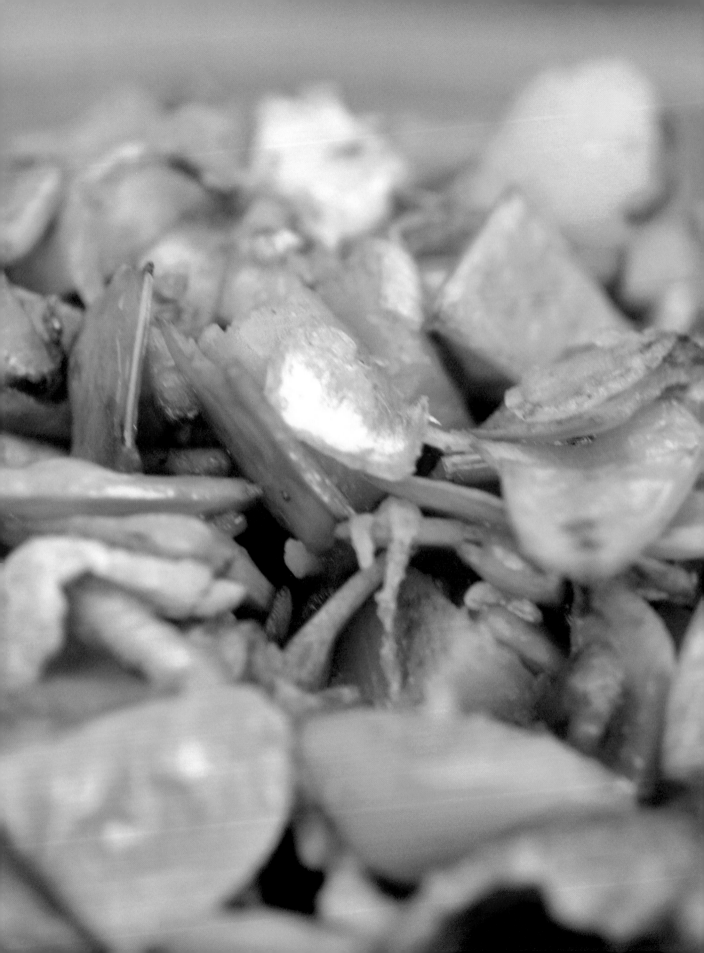

Hearty mix

- Peel and chop the sweet potato into cubes and boil in a small saucepan until cooked through

- Add the olive oil to a frying pan and fry the bacon on low to medium heat

- Once crispy, remove from the pan and set aside

- Chop an onion and add to the pan

- Sautee the onion until it starts to show a golden hint, then add roughly chopped mange tout and sweet peas and the sweet potato

- After a few minutes, add the chopped bacon and a pinch of salt

- Cook through on a low heat

- Have your bowl at the ready and once cooked through serve immediately

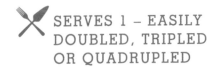

SERVES 1 – EASILY DOUBLED, TRIPLED OR QUADRUPLED

Handful mange tout and sweet peas

1 onion

2 rashers bacon

Pinch coarse sea salt

½ sweet potato

2 tablespoons olive oil

Sprinkling of parmesan (optional)

57

This is one of those light speedy meals that came together as a product of being tired after a long day, having absolutely nothing in the fridge and needing a nutritious meal, involving as little creativity and finesse as possible. Incredibly simple, unadulterated flavours.

I'm a big fan of burgers. Not the dry, crumbly ones or indeed the hockey puck ones with the potential to take out an eye, but rather moist, meaty burgers with a subtle but juicy flavour. Being Polish, my Babcia (grandmother) makes amazing kotlety – the polish equivalent to the traditional beef burger. Normally these burgers are coated in a layer of breadcrumbs to seal in the moisture. However, here, I've adapted the recipe to make the mini burgers I love so much!

58

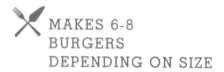

MAKES 6-8 BURGERS DEPENDING ON SIZE

500g pork mince

2 onions

½ teaspoon white pepper

1 teaspoon coarse sea salt

Handful ground almonds

Oil of your choice

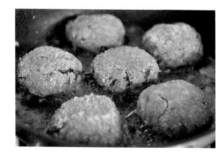

Burgers

- Chop the onion as finely as possible and with a generous splash of oil, add to a frying pan on low heat; don't be tempted to fry on a higher heat, as the onion will end up being too crunchy and sharp tasting in the burgers

- Once the onion has turned golden and slightly brown at the edges, remove from the heat and add to the mince, along with the white pepper and salt, using your hands to mix the ingredients

- Form the mince into balls and flatten slightly, forming a burger shape

- Coat the burger in ground almonds

- In the frying pan, on medium heat, add enough oil to cover halfway up the burgers

- Add the burgers to the pan

- Once the burgers are cooked three quarters of the way up (the timing depends on the size of your burgers) flip them over to cook the other side

- Check the burgers are cooked through by cutting one in half. They should not have any pink or red in the middle

- Once they are cooked through, remove them from the pan and serve them on their own or in a bun with sweet potato fries and tomato ketchup

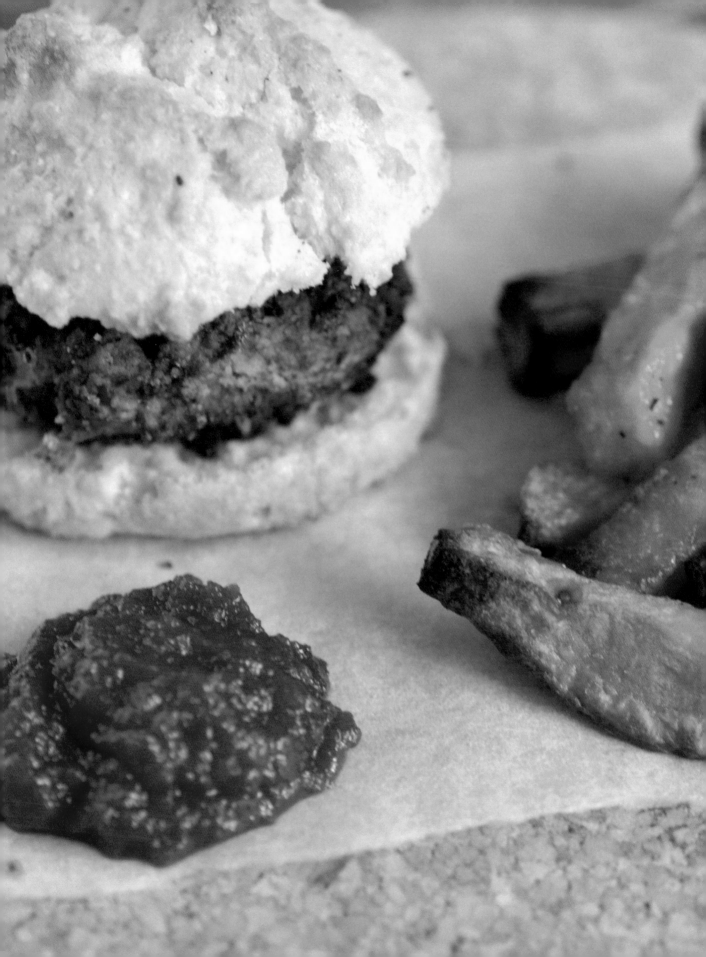

Some recipes take more than a couple of test runs to earn a place in my personal recipe stash but making this for the first time was a resounding success. One bite of the mixed spice infused duck on a bed of wilted spinach, drenched in the resulting jus and my family were hooked.

Pan fried duck breast, spinach and the most amazing roux

SERVES 2

2 duck breasts

1 tablespoon olive oil

2 tablespoons balsamic vinegar

Coarse sea salt

Black pepper

1 teaspoon ground mixed spice

2 large handfuls spinach

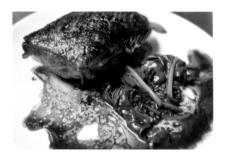

- Heat the olive oil and balsamic vinegar with a pinch of salt in a frying pan on a medium heat

- In a crisscross pattern, score the skin side of the duck breasts

- Mix the ground mixed spice, salt and pepper and rub all over the duck breasts

- Once the pan is hot, add the duck breasts, skin side down

- Allow to cook for a few minutes on medium heat, then turn the heat down to cook for a further 15 minutes until the skin is brown and crispy

- Flip the duck breasts over and continue to cook for approximately 10 minutes to leave a slight pink tinge in the middle of the breast – timing depends on the size of the duck breasts and how well done you like your meat. So cook for a shorter or longer time depending on your preferences.

- Add the spinach to the pan and turn off the heat, allowing the spinach to sauté in the hot jus

- Once cooked to your liking, serve the duck breasts either whole or sliced on a plate on top of the spinach with the jus poured over

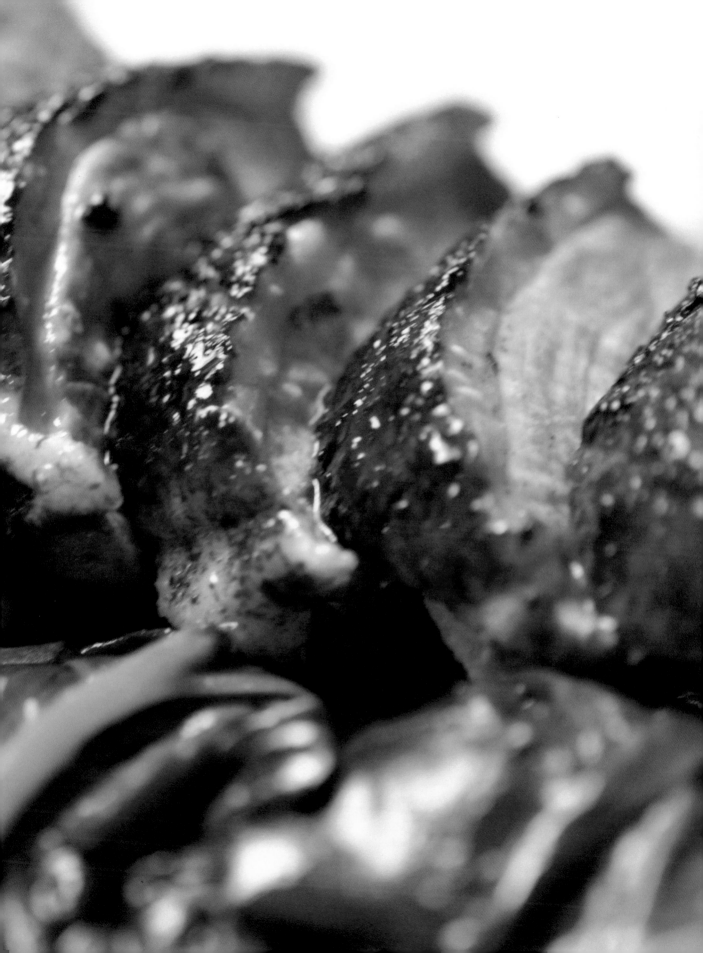

I personally don't see the point in eating curries with a spiciness so hot, it feels like your tongue's about to drop off. I'd much prefer to be able to taste the flavours and savour the meal without having to keep in mind the nearest location of a jug of water whilst trying to get through the meal, eyes watering and turning a significantly darker shade of red. This curry is more my style, mildly spiced with a creamy thick coconut milk texture.

62

SERVES 2

1 onion

1 leek

2 tablespoons walnut oil

¾ teaspoon coarse sea salt

¾ teaspoon garam marsala

⅛ teaspoon ginger

Pinch cayenne pepper

¾ teaspoon coriander

¾ teaspoon cumin

500g lamb mince

400ml coconut milk

3 tablespoons tomato puree

1 handful spinach

Lamb curry

- Heat the walnut oil in a frying pan on low heat

- Chop the onion and leek and add to the pan, stirring occasionally until the onion turns soft and starts turning golden brown round the edges

- Remove from the pan and set aside until later

- Turn the heat up and add the lamb mince to the pan

- Brown the mince, breaking it up and stirring occasionally

- Add the salt, garam marsala, ginger, cayenne pepper, coriander and cumin to the pan and stir

- Add the tomato puree and coconut milk

- Bring to the boil and give the contents a stir

- Boil for a few minutes and then turn the heat down to low, placing a lid on the pan and continue to simmer for 40 minutes – add small amounts of water if the curry starts to become too dry

- Once cooked, stir in the spinach and remove from the heat

- Serve whilst still hot, over bowls of cauliflower rice

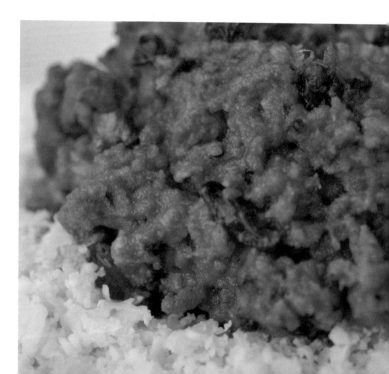

Cheesy risotto

Ok, so it's not exactly a spitting image of risotto but this cheesy comforting dish makes a good stand in for the real thing. Full of taste, making a filling bowlful without being too heavy.

- Sauté the onion in the walnut oil in a frying pan on a low heat

- Grate the cauliflower and once the onion and leek are tuning golden brown, add to the pan

- Continue to sauté the cauliflower for a minute or two before adding the water to the pan; the mixture may look watery but the water will boil off as it simmers

- Allow to simmer for approximately 5 minutes before adding grated cheddar cheese and the parmesan cheese

- Stir whilst the cheese melts, binding the mixture together

- Once the cheese has melted and the mixture has come together and thickened, add the cream and give a stir before adding a few chopped chives and serving

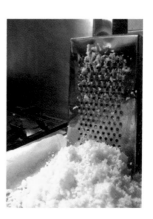

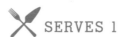 SERVES 1

2 tablespoons walnut oil

1 onion

1 small leek

Sea salt

Black pepper

50g cheddar cheese

150ml water

½ head cauliflower

Large handful parmesan cheese

2 tablespoons cream (optional)

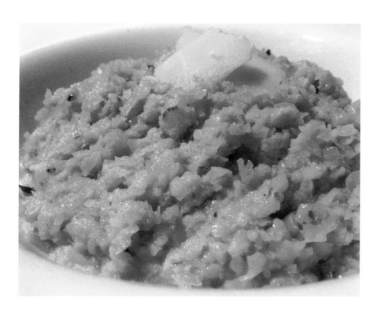

Sea bass has such a delicate flavour, simple seasoning is all that's needed to bring out its mouth-watering natural flavour.

Lemon Sea Bass with Asparagus

- Chop a centimetre or two off the end of the asparagus stalks and add to a frying pan with a splash of oil on a low to medium heat

- Fry the asparagus with salt for approximately 10 minutes

- Add a splash of oil to a frying pan on medium heat

- Add the sea bass fillet, skin side down with salt and black pepper to taste and fry for 2-3 minutes or until the fillet starts to cook, turning white round the edges

- Turn the fillet to cook on the other side for a minute or until the fillet is just cooked through

- Chop the lemon in half and squeeze lemon juice over the fillet

SERVES 2

2 fillets sea bass

Black pepper

Sea salt

350g asparagus spears

1 lemon

64

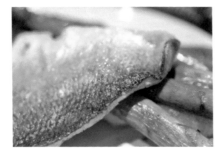

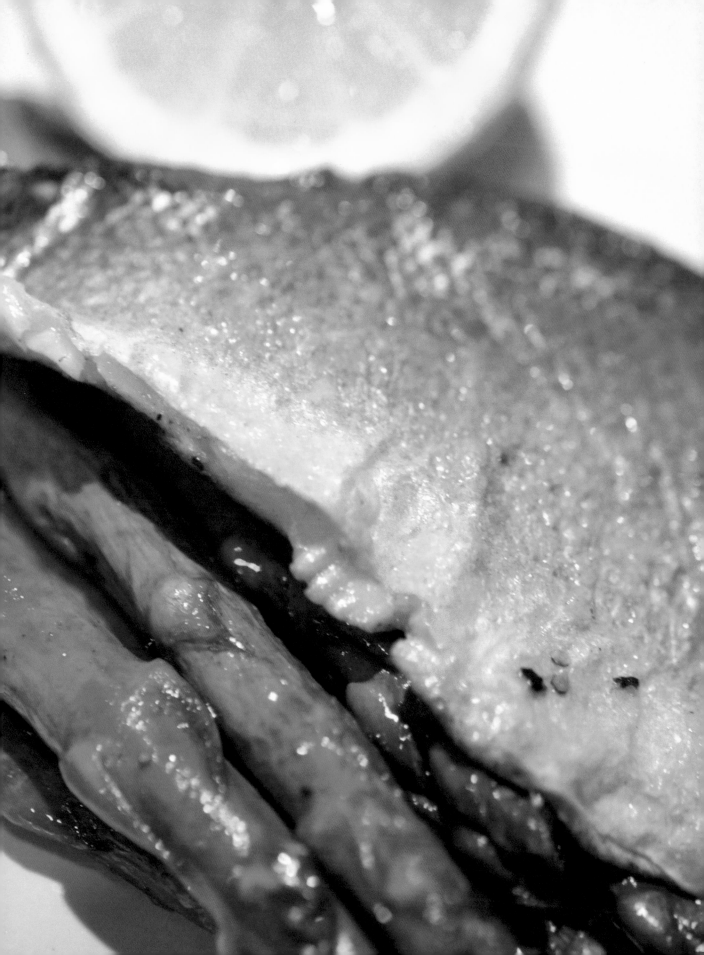

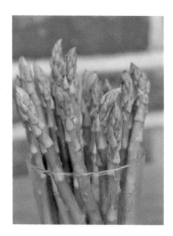

Roast chicken, asparagus spears and plum tomato casserole

✕ SERVES 4

4 chicken legs

200g plum tomatoes

1 large bunch asparagus

Olive oil

Butter

2 tablespoons thyme

¼ teaspoon coarse sea salt

Black pepper

40ml lemon juice

400ml water

1 bag bouquet garni

50ml double cream

- Preheat the oven to 180 degrees celsius (fan assisted oven)

- In a frying pan on high heat, brown the chicken legs in olive oil and butter – approximately 2 minutes each side

- Once browned, add the chicken legs to a casserole dish

- In the frying pan, reduce to a medium heat and lightly sauté the asparagus before adding it to the casserole dish

- Wash and halve the baby plum tomatoes and add in to the dish, along with the thyme, sea salt, black pepper, lemon juice, water, bouquet garni bag and the double cream

- Place the casserole lid over the dish (or cover with foil) and place in the oven for approximately 1 hour and 20 minutes or until the chicken is cooked through

- Once cooked, remove from the oven and taste, removing the bouquet garni bag and adding any extra salt needed before serving

❛ Chicken legs are an easy staple to have handy. Place the chicken legs inside a foil lined baking dish with salt, pepper and olive oil and cover over with a second piece of foil. Bake 4 legs for an hour in a preheated oven at 180 degrees celsius (fan assisted oven) and then uncover the second piece of foil for a further 20 minutes to make the skin crispy and golden. You can drain off any resulting juices in the bottom of the dish and add to give a stock or soup a deeper flavour. Wrap the legs up and store in the fridge, picking at them for snacks or tearing off the meat and throwing them on a salad or in a dish like my chicken satay recipe. However, to make things a bit more exciting, I sometimes make this slightly more elaborate chicken dish. The stock from the chicken seeps into the sauce, giving a more intense flavour. ❜

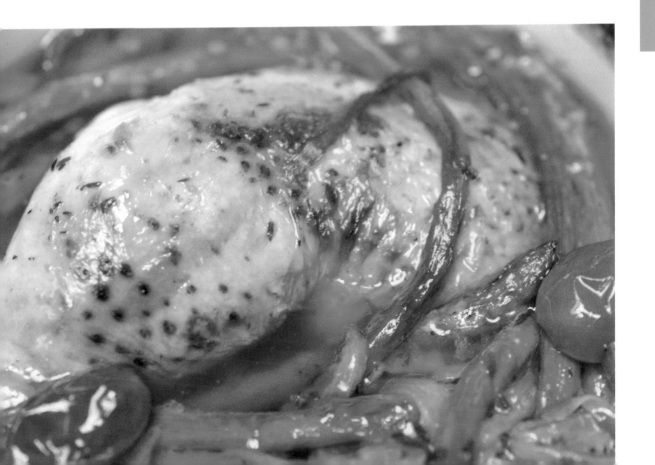

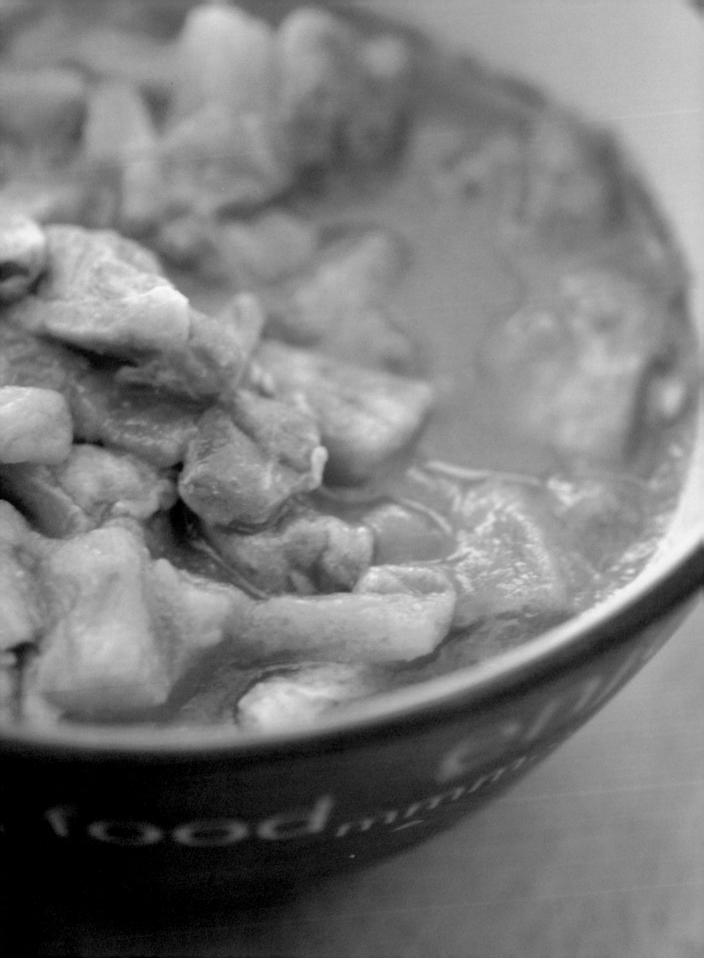

On my last few trips into town before getting very unwell, I discovered sweet and sour chicken. On my way back home I would stop off at the takeaway and walk back home munching on a large box of sticky white rice and super sweet, sweet and sour chicken. Unfortunately most sweet and sour chicken often comes with a hefty sugar and soy dose, but not this one.

Sweet and sour chicken

- Add the walnut oil to a frying pan on medium heat
- Chop the chicken thighs into small chunks and add to the pan along with the ginger, salt and white pepper
- Fry the chicken until cooked through
- Add the tomato puree, honey, balsamic vinegar, white wine vinegar, water, pineapple juice and pineapple chunks
- Bring to the boil and then turn down the heat and allow to simmer
- Add the coconut flour gradually, stirring in between additions to reach a thicker consistency
- Once heated through, serve with a side of cauli rice or over stir fried vegetables

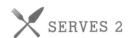 SERVES 2

4 chicken thighs

2 tablespoons walnut oil

1 tablespoon tomato puree

30ml white wine vinegar

Couple pinches of salt

2 tablespoons honey

50ml water

1 tablespoon balsamic vinegar

¼ teaspoon ginger

⅛ teaspoon white pepper

1½ tablespoons coconut flour

220g of pineapple chunks and pineapple juice

69

I'm a huge fan of paninis and flat breads rather than stodgy sandwiches consisting of 90% bread, hiding away a measly amount of filling. I think of the bread component as more of a vehicle for the tasty filling. In this way quesadillas are great. Being thin, they are light and you can really concentrate on the scrumptious fillings, which is, let's be honest, the really interesting bit, yet still have the convenience of holding it together in a sandwich form, making them great for trips or quick lunches. Or even make a couple of different fillings and pack to take on a picnic! I can't say enough about these!

Quesadillas

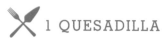 1 QUESADILLA

One wrap recipe (see beautiful basics)

Splash of oil for frying

Half a yellow pepper

Chives

Ham

Small handful of cheddar cheese

- Make one of my wraps, as detailed earlier in the book

- Slice thin strips of the yellow pepper and sauté in olive oil on a low heat until soft

- Lay the wrap out flat on the work surface

- On one side of the wrap layer the ham, yellow peppers and chopped chives, finally sprinkling cheddar cheese over the top

- Fold the other side of the wrap over the layers so your wrap is folded in half, with the filling sandwiched inside

- Place the folded wrap in a frying pan on a medium heat and cook for 5 minutes on both sides or until the outside is golden brown and the cheese has melted, sticking the wrap together

- Remove the quesadilla from the pan and cut in half

- Wrap each half in a piece of kitchen roll or greaseproof paper so you can easily hold and eat whilst still warm

70

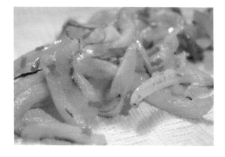

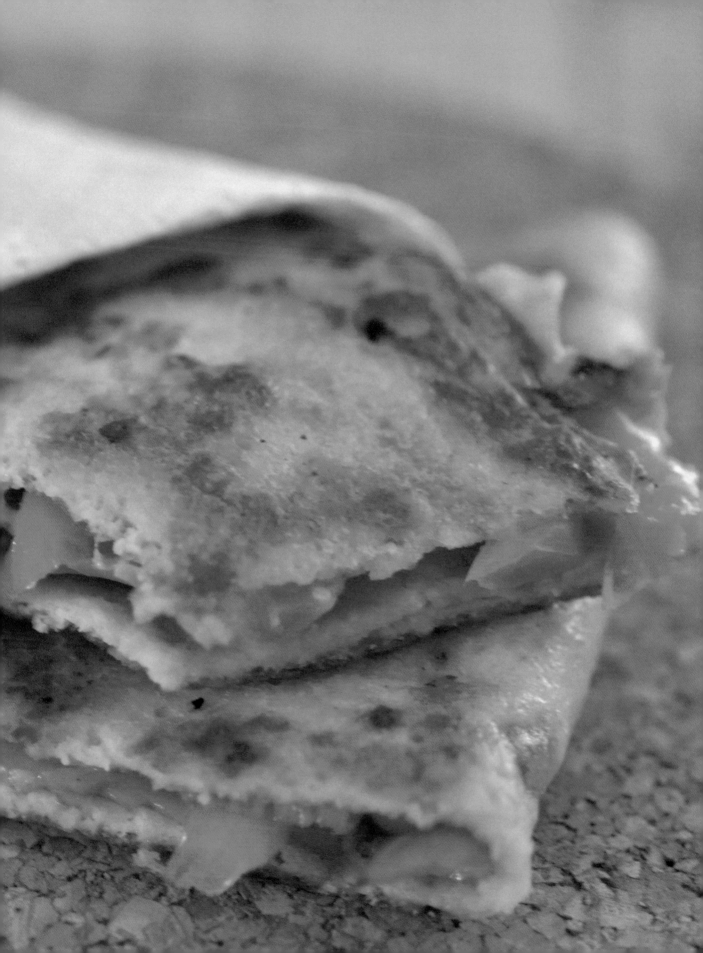

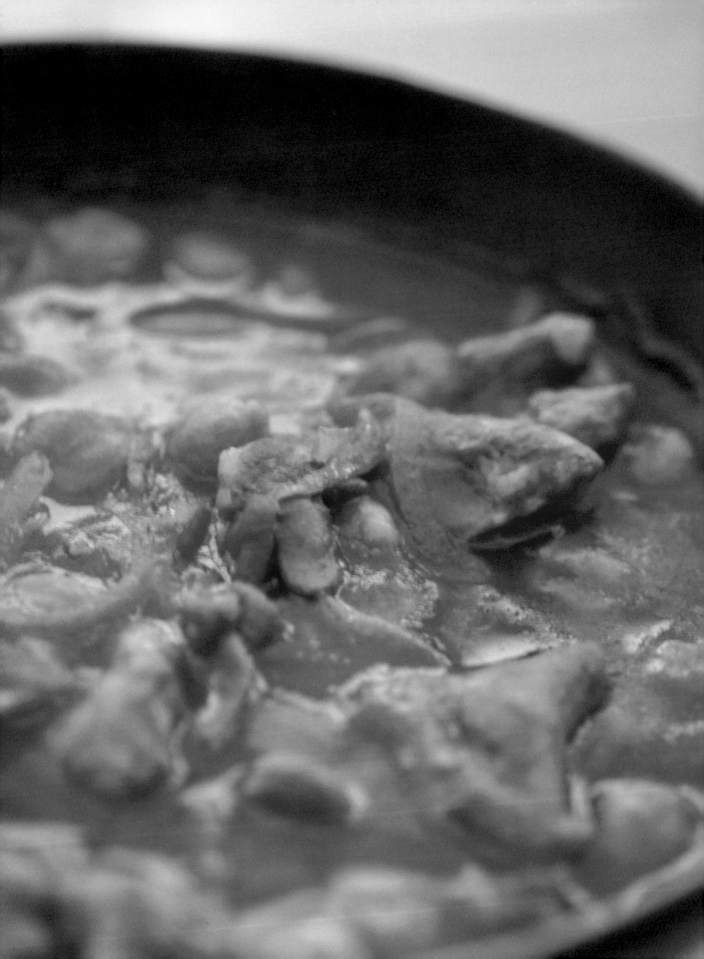

A more everyday meal, make this dish on a weekday after a long day of work to replenish your energy stores.

Bacon, chicken and chickpea pot

- Fry the rashers of bacon in a frying pan on a low to medium heat

- Once cooked and crispy, remove the bacon from the pan and set aside

- Heat the coconut oil in a saucepan on a medium heat

- Cut the chicken thighs into thin strips and brown in the pan with a finely chopped onion, salt and white pepper

- Once the chicken is browned, add the chicken stock, tomato passata and bouquet garni to the pan

- Bring to the boil for 2 minutes

- Place the lid over the pan to cover and reduce to a simmer for 20-30 minutes or until the chicken is cooked through

- Chop the bacon pieces and add to the pan with the cooked chickpeas

- Simmer for another 5 minutes and serve

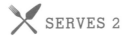 SERVES 2

1 onion

3 rashers bacon

4 chicken thighs

1 tablespoon coconut oil

¼ teaspoon white pepper

¼ teaspoon salt

300ml chicken stock

200ml tomato passata

1 bouquet garni

150g cooked chickpeas

73

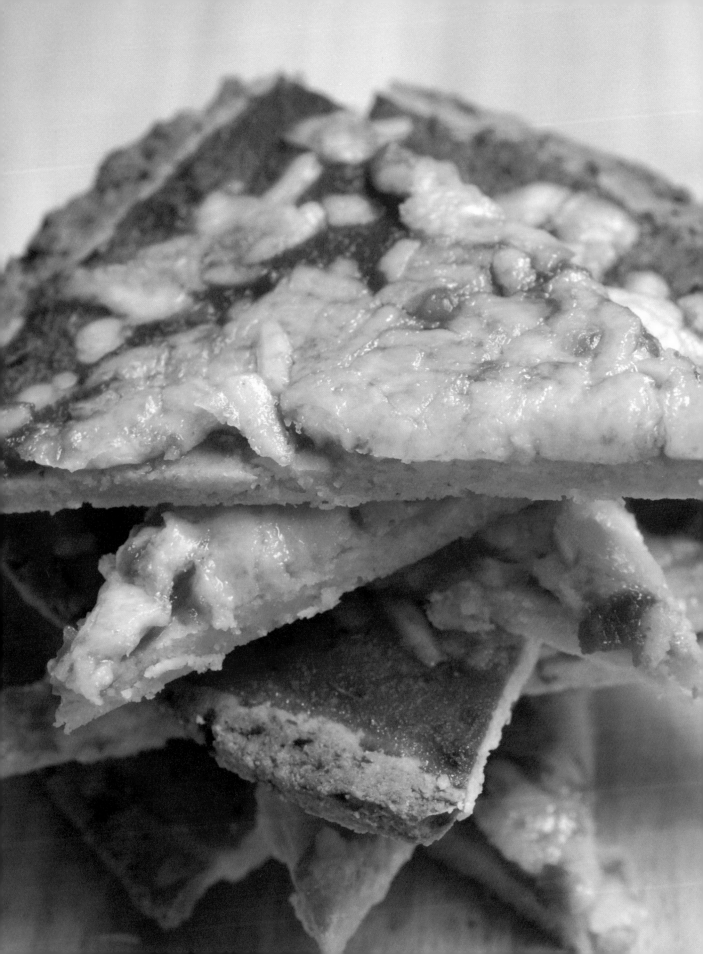

When I was younger our family went through a phase of ordering a takeaway pizza most Friday nights. After watching how some of the fast food chains handle the food, our appetite for takeaways seemed to abandon us and we decided to make our own pizzas at home or buy better quality pizzas. Omitting grains also means omitting pizza. Right? Not a chance. Here's the pizza we turn to when craving a slice.

Pizza

- Preheat oven to 170 degrees celsius (fan assisted oven)

- Add egg whites, salt and cream cheese in a bowl and mix

- Add the ground almonds and mix in well

- Line a baking sheet with a sheet of greaseproof paper

- Spread out the mixture over the greaseproof sheet, making a circular shape and place in the oven for 10 minutes or until the base is firm and starting to show a bit of colour

- Remove the pizza base from the oven and leave to cool

- Once cooled, spread the tomato sauce over the base and then sprinkle cheese, plus any other toppings to finish and place back in the oven until the cheese starts bubbling

- Remove from the oven and leave to cool slightly before slicing and serving

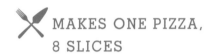 MAKES ONE PIZZA, 8 SLICES

100g ground almonds

1 egg white

Salt

2 tablespoons low fat cream cheese

1 tomato sauce recipe or the quick tomato sauce used on my omelette pizza

Large handful or two of cheddar cheese plus any additional toppings

75

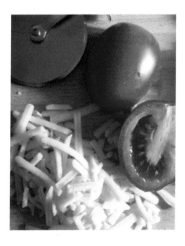

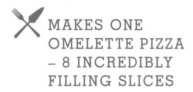

**MAKES ONE
OMELETTE PIZZA
– 8 INCREDIBLY
FILLING SLICES**

2 large handfuls spinach

Pinch sea salt

A blob of butter

Splash of olive oil

6 egg whites (or 4 whole eggs)

75g cheddar cheese

50g walnuts

76

Omelette pizza

- Preheat a grill to 190 degrees celsius

- Add the butter and olive oil to a skillet on low to medium heat

- Tear the spinach and add to the pan

- Finely chop the walnuts and grate 50g of the cheese. Add these to the pan

- Add the salt and stir

- When the cheese starts to melt, whisk your egg whites or eggs briefly until slightly frothy and add to the pan

- Quickly give the contents of the pan a quick stir to mix together all the ingredients, before the egg gets a chance to cook

- Allow the egg to cook through for about 5 minutes or until the circle is fairly firm, only leaving the surface of the omelette uncooked

- Place the skillet under the grill for about 3 minutes or until the top of the omelette has just about cooked

- Remove the omelette from the grill and spread tomato sauce over the top of the omelette

- Grate 25g of the remaining cheddar cheese and sprinkle over the top

- Place back under the grill for another 5 minutes or until the cheese has melted and starts to bubble

- Remove from the grill and allow to cool slightly before sliding the omelette pizza onto a chopping board and cutting into slices

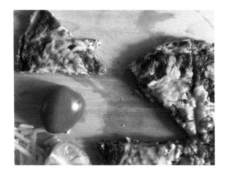

For those of you wanting a substitute for a pizza, completely true to its aesthetic form and taste I have included a pizza recipe made with a savoury almond base. Yet I felt compelled to include another option. Most mornings I will have eggs and good quality bacon or some kind of omelette. Having a bit of a thing for the pizza taste, and not wanting to eat baked goods with a nut base all the time, I am more than happy to make my monster of an omelette pizza. Filling is an understatement and I can usually manage no more than half this omelette pizza tops. Usually I can leave the left overs on the counter and someone will no doubt come along and finish the job for me. In the rare cases in which you find yourself with leftovers, store surplus slices in the fridge for snacking or take into work for a lunch.

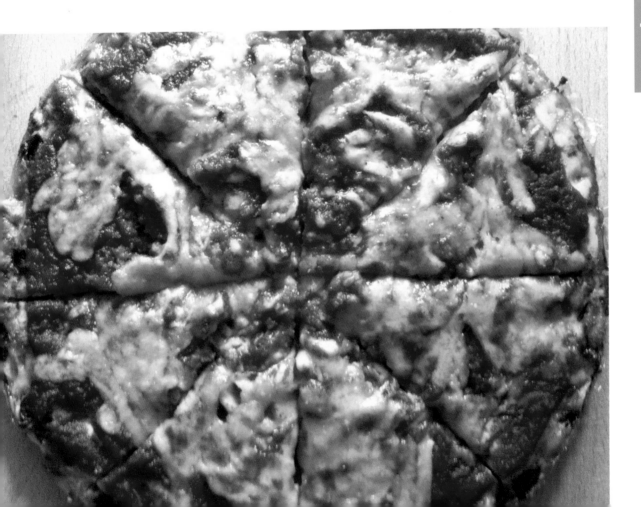

> *A different tomato sauce is used for the almond based pizza, however, when making this omelette, it's usually time for breakfast and being impatient, I'm usually looking for the quickest, least fussy option, so I throw together this super quick sauce.*

SERVES 2

100ml tomato passata

½ teaspoon oregano

Pinch white pepper

Large pinch salt

Quick tomato sauce

- Mix all ingredients together in a small bowl
- Pour and spread out over omelette pizza

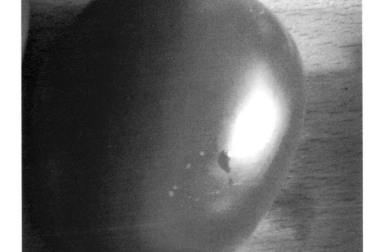

Stewed beef

- Heat the olive oil in a saucepan on medium heat
- When the pan is hot, add the stewing beef and brown the meat
- When the meat is completely browned on the outside, add the water to the pan
- Add the tomato puree, salt, pepper and bouquet garni and bring to the boil for 5 minutes before reducing the heat
- Replace the saucepan lid and leave to simmer for 4-5 hours occasionally stirring and adding small amounts of water if the liquid level is too low
- The beef will be done when the meat easily tears
- When the beef is cooked, remove from the heat
- Before serving locate the bouquet garni bag and remove this before serving with a side of cauli mash

Slow cooking the beef means the meat just falls apart. As an added bonus, no stock needs to be added as the beef juices add to the water and seasonings, creating a stock and rich gravy all at once.

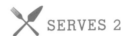 SERVES 2

500g stewing beef

500ml water

2½ tablespoons tomato puree

½ teaspoon coarse sea salt

Large pinch white pepper

1 bouquet garni bag

Splash olive oil

79

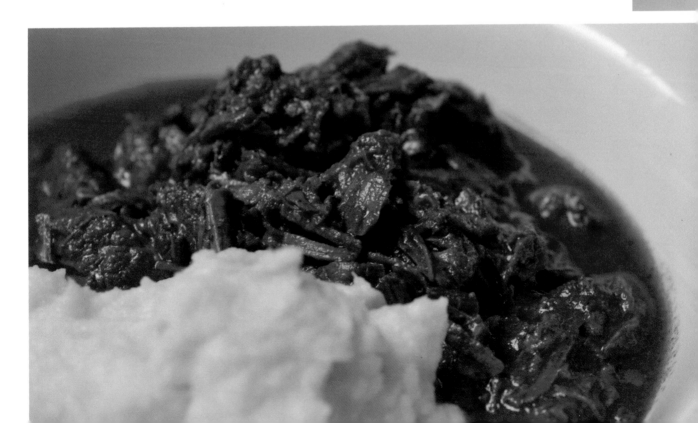

SIDES CAN DOMINATE A MEAL. CHIPS
CAN OVERPOWER A PUB LUNCH AND
SPAGHETTI BOLOGNAISE CONSISTS,
MORE OFTEN THAN NOT, OF A MERE
SPOONFUL OF BOLOGNAISE PERCHING
ATOP AN INSURMOUNTABLE MOUNTAIN
OF SPAGHETTI. INSTEAD OF FILLING UP
ON NUTRITIONALLY DEVOID SIDES, MAKE
ONE OF THESE AS AN ACCOMPANIMENT TO
YOUR MAIN DISH OR EVEN SERVE AS A MAIN
DISH IN ITSELF FOR A LIGHT MEAL

succulent
sides & salads

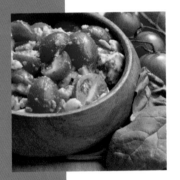

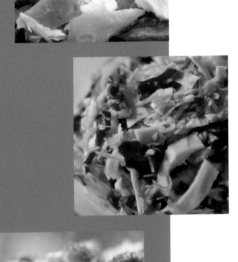

⁶ To do this salad justice use in season berries to make this sweet and nutty summer salad. ⁹

Strawberry salad

- Wash and chop the strawberries

- Wash and tear up the spinach leaves

- Place all ingredients in a salad bowl and sprinkle over the hazelnuts

- Add the balsamic-hazelnut vinaigrette and serve in a small bowl on the side

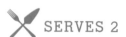 SERVES 2

150g strawberries

2 handfuls spinach

Small handful of chopped hazelnuts

Balsamic-hazelnut vinaigrette

82

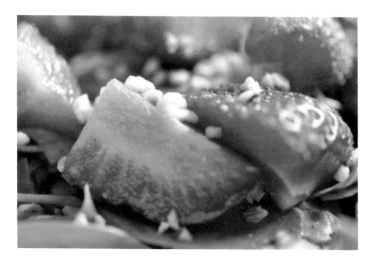

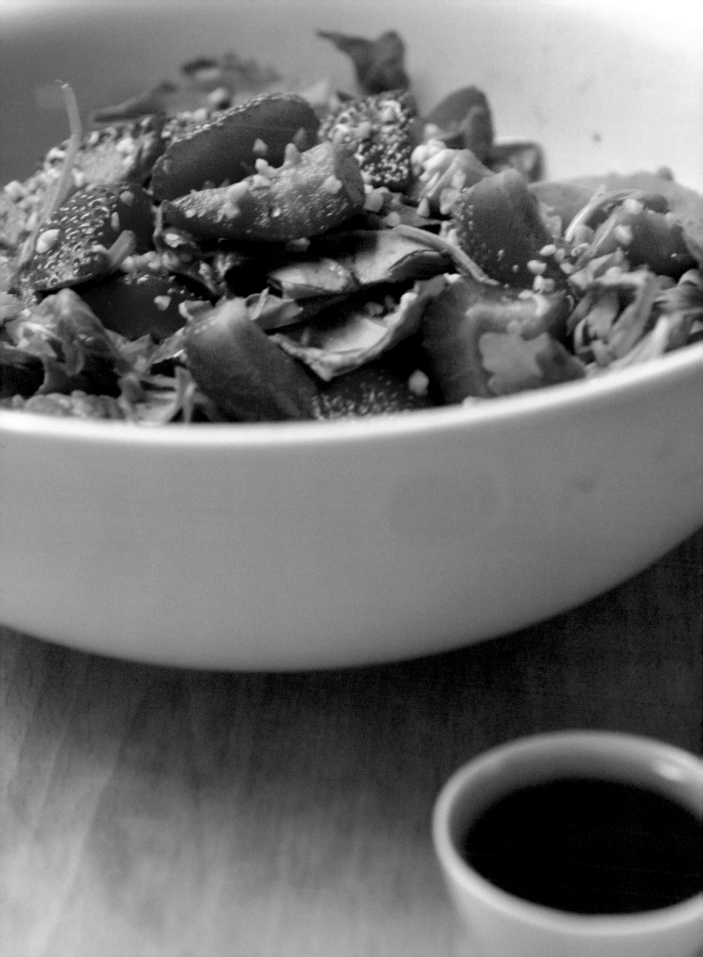

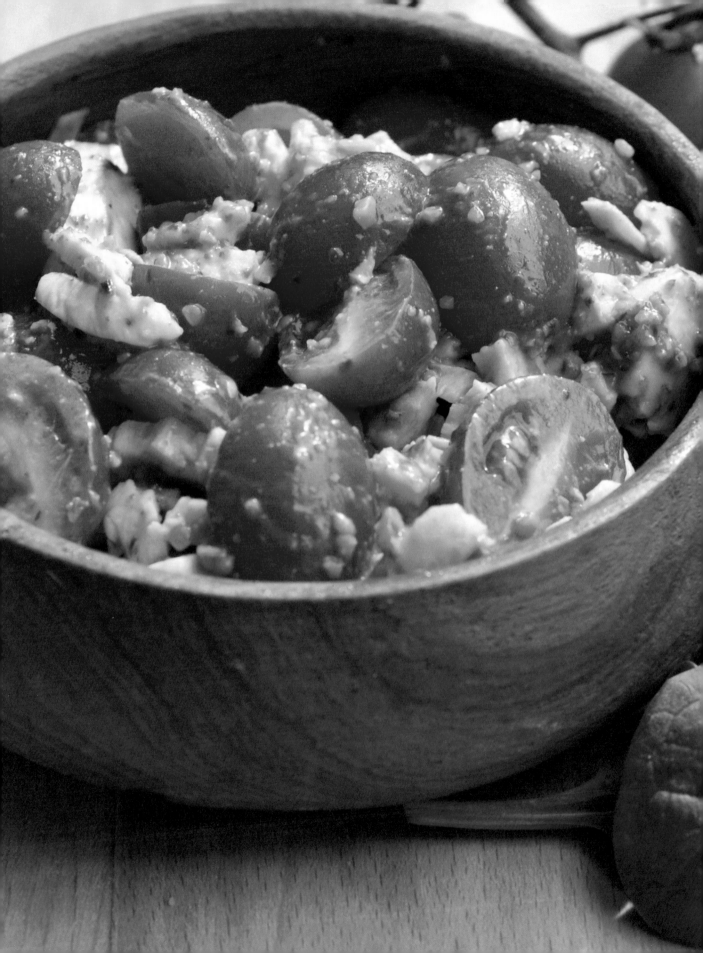

Tomato, mozzarella, pesto salad

- Wash and chop the tomatoes in half

- Use your fingers to tear the mozzarella into smaller chunks

- Add all the tomato halves and mozzarella pieces to a bowl

- Spoon the pesto over the top and give a quick mix to give an even covering of pesto

- Chop the chives and scatter over the top of the salad to serve

Wonderfully fresh, rustic salad.

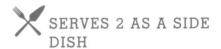

SERVES 2 AS A SIDE DISH

6 baby plum tomatoes

1 ball mozzarella

1 generously heaped tablespoon pesto

A few chives

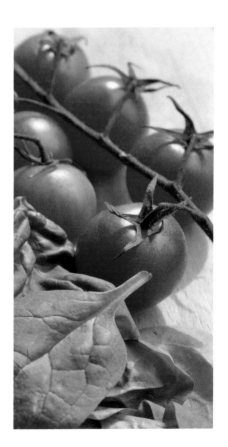

85

A light, fresh salmon salad.

Light salmon salad

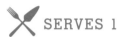

SERVES 1

1 salmon fillet

100g green dwarf beans

6 baby new potatoes

1 mayonnaise recipe (see mmm...saucy)

Dill

Chives

Sea salt

Black pepper

- Wash and chop the new potatoes into cubes

- Boil the new potatoes in water with a pinch of salt

- Add the green dwarf beans to the saucepan once the potatoes are almost cooked

- Continue to boil for another 3 minutes or until the potatoes and green dwarf beans are cooked

- Once cooked, drain the water and set aside the potatoes and green beans to cool

- Add a splash of oil to a frying pan on medium heat

- Add the salmon fillet, skin side down with salt and black pepper and fry for 5 minutes or until there is a colour change a third of the way up the fillet

- Turn the fillet to cook on the other side for a few minutes, until the fillet is cooked through

- Make the mayonnaise and add to the cooled potatoes and green beans along with chopped fresh chives, dill and salt and pepper to taste

- Either place the whole salmon fillet at the side of the potato and green bean salad or flake the fillet in, mix together and serve

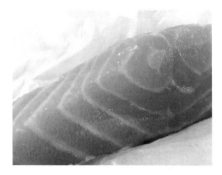

Butter beans, tomato and parmesan

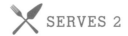
An easy and tasty side to most meals.

- Preheat the oven to 200 degrees celsius (fan assisted oven)

- Place the butter beans into a shallow baking dish along with the chopped tomatoes, black pepper, salt, oregano, basil and olive oil

- Mix all the ingredients together

- Sprinkle the grated parmesan cheese evenly over the top of the beans and place in the oven for approximately 15 - 20 minutes or until the cheese has melted and begins to bubble

- Once cooked, remove from the oven and serve whilst still warm

SERVES 2

230g cooked butter beans

400g carton chopped tomatoes

Black pepper

2 pinches of coarse sea salt

½ teaspoon oregano

½ teaspoon basil

1 tablespoon olive oil

2 handfuls parmesan

87

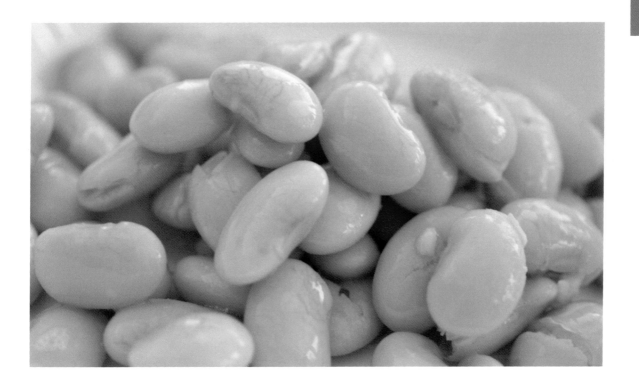

The slightly salty ham and the sweet mango give a lovely contrast of simple flavours.

Ham, mango and mozzarella salad

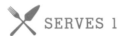 SERVES 1

½ mango

4 slices ham

½ ball mozzerella

Handful of walnuts

Drizzle olive oil

2 large handfuls of leaves
(I like any combination of
romaine, rocket, watercress
and frisee)

2 slices prosciutto

Pinch of sea salt

- Tear the leaves, ham and mozzarella into pieces

- Peel half a mango and chop the flesh into small cubes

- Roughly chop a handful of walnuts

- Add all ingredients to a salad bowl and drizzle olive oil over the top to dress with a pinch of salt

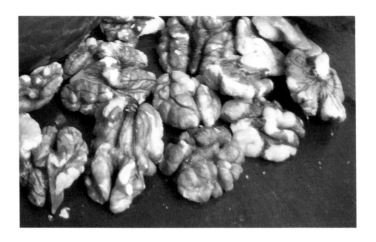

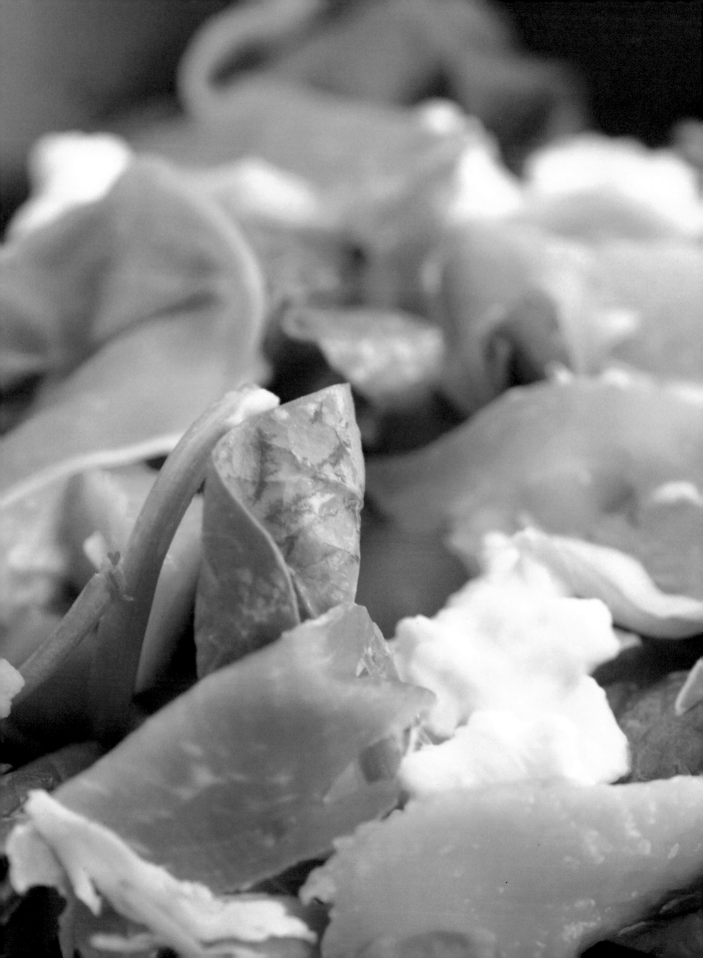

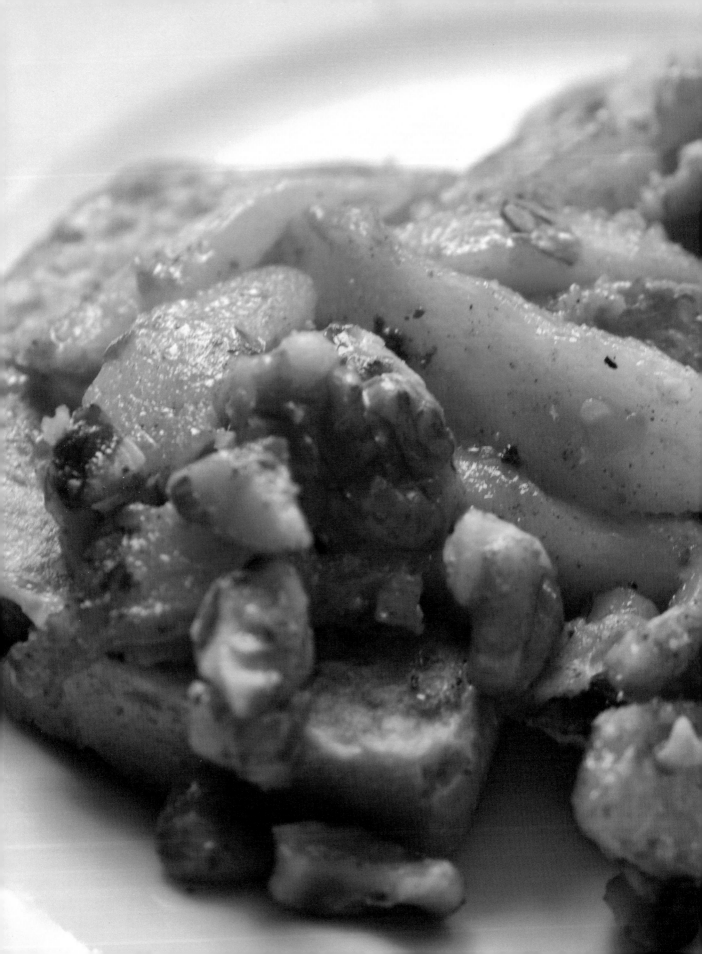

Pear and walnut with eggy bread

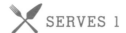
Not at all complicated, this quick meal is fresh and perfect for a light lunch.

Make the eggy bread;

- Crack the egg into a shallow but wide bowl

- Add the salt and cinnamon and whisk the egg mixture with a fork

- Dunk the two slices of bread into the egg, covering both sides in the egg mixture

- Heat a splash of oil or a knob of butter in a frying pan on medium heat

- Once heated, add the bread slices to the pan

- Fry until the egg has set on one side of the bread and then flip the bread over to cook the other side

- Once nicely fried on both sides, remove from the pan and place on a plate

Sauté the pear;

- Peel and slice the pear into thin slices

- Grind a small pinch of black pepper, a pinch of salt and a generous drizzle of walnut oil into a frying pan on a low heat

- Add the pear to the frying pan and allow to sauté

- Add some roughly crushed walnuts, moving the pears occasionally

- Once the pears are slightly softened and browned, remove from the heat and serve the pears and walnut pieces over the eggy bread

SERVES 1

1 egg

Pinch of sea salt

2 slices of bread
(see beautiful basics)

Small pinch of cinnamon

1 pear

Black pepper

Splash of walnut oil

A small handful of walnuts

Large pinch coarse sea salt

91

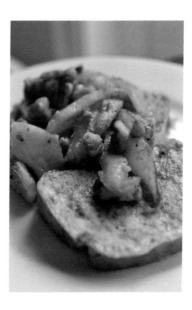

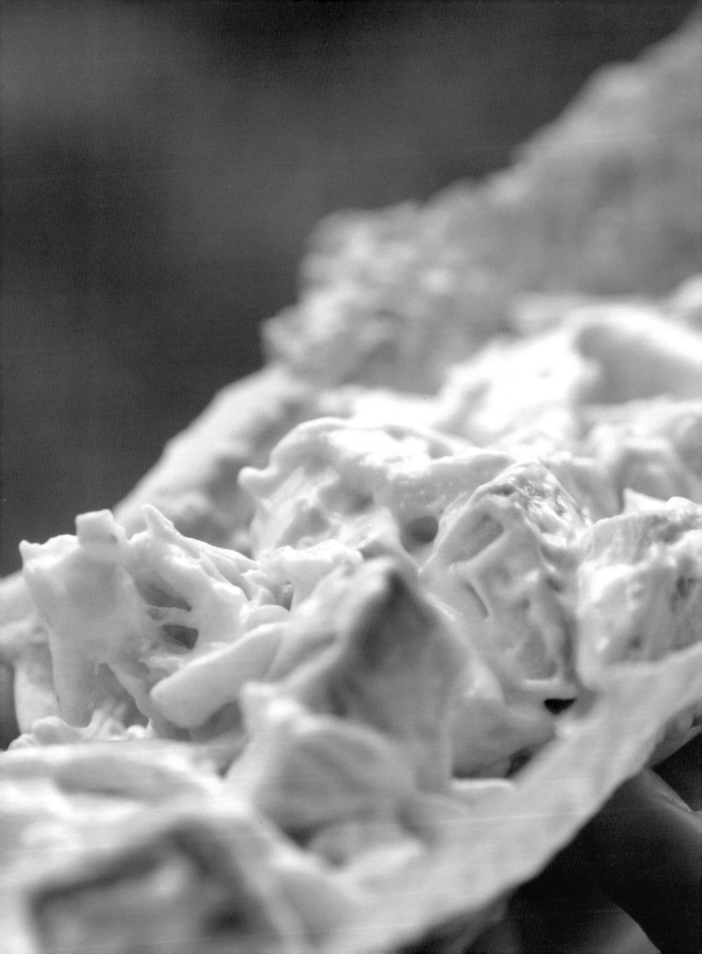

Without a heavy, stodgy bread component, the filling in these lettuce boats becomes the main focus and as we all know, the filling's always the best part of a sandwich anyway!

Avocado and chicken mayonnaise boats

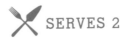

SERVES 2

A couple of romaine lettuce leaves

1 avocado

1 mayonnaise recipe (see mmm...saucy)

Chives

2 handfuls of cooked chicken

Sea salt

- Peel and chop the avocado into cubes and add to a bowl along with chopped chives, the mayonnaise and the torn cooked chicken

- Mix together all the ingredients in the bowl and add salt to taste

- Spoon the mixture into the lettuce leaves

- Serve

93

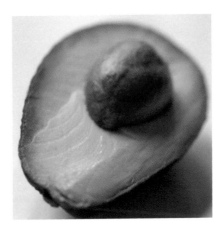

Moist, cheesy and full of flavour, this bread is as far as you can get from ordinary, dry, tasteless bread. Perfect for tearing and sharing.

Tabletop bread

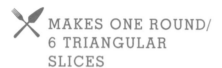

MAKES ONE ROUND/
6 TRIANGULAR
SLICES

100g cauliflower

75g ground almonds

2 egg whites

25g butter

Pinch white pepper

Pinch sea salt

1 teaspoon thyme

½ teaspoon bicarbonate of soda

25g cheddar cheese – plus a handful for topping

- Steam the cauliflower until soft. If you don't own a steamer, then use a small saucepan with a small volume of water in the bottom. Boil the water, and place the lid on the saucepan and reduce the heat to a simmer. Keep an eye on the volume of water in the saucepan and add a splash or two if the level diminishes

- Once the cauliflower is cooked through and soft, puree using a hand blender

- Leave the cauliflower puree to one side to cool

- Preheat the oven to 170 degrees celsius (fan assisted oven)

- In a mixing bowl add the ground almonds, butter, egg whites, white pepper, sea salt, thyme, ½ teaspoon bicarbonate of soda and 25g grated cheddar cheese and using a spoon, mix together

- Once the cauliflower has cooled, add the puree to the mixture and mix in

- Spoon the mixture into a heap onto a greaseproof paper lined baking tray

- Spread the mixture into a circular shape about 2cm thick or an oblong shape for a longer bread

- Place in the oven for approximately 10-15 minutes

- Remove from the oven once the round has colour and turns golden brown round the edges and the cheese has melted. The centre should be slightly moist so the outside will not be firm

- Once removed from the oven leave to cool for 10-20 minutes before cutting into slices

94

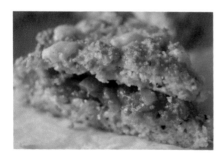

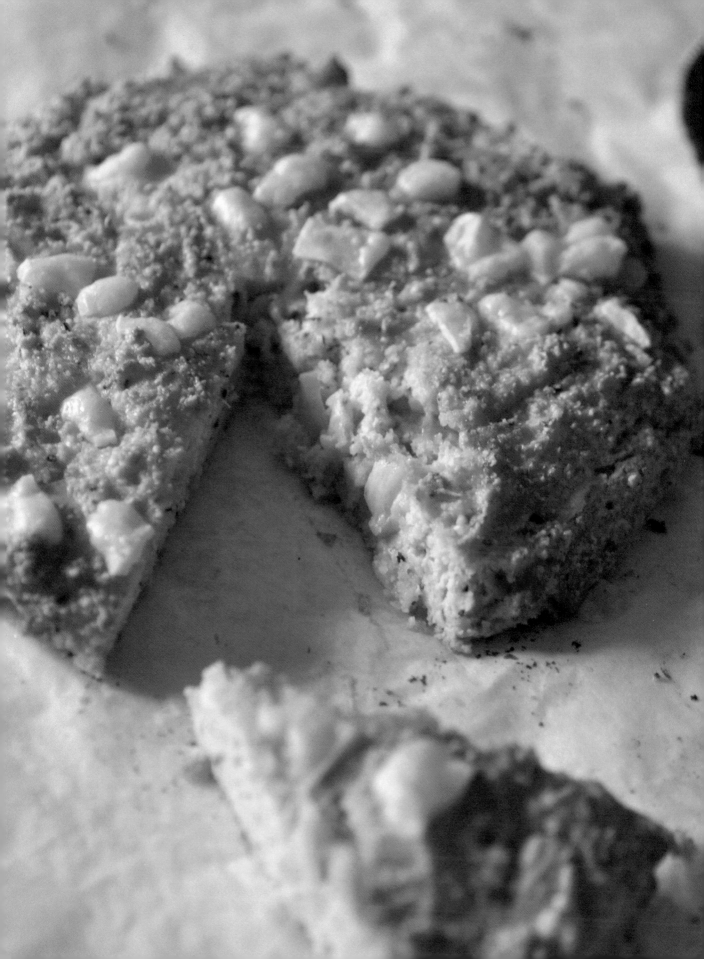

In England we love our traditional mash. However the average potato mash can be a heavy, high GI component to a meal. I'm a big fan of using a diverse range of vegetables in as many dishes as possible, so cauliflower steamed and pureed can be used to create a lighter mash. Add seasoning to your taste or make it even more interesting with other flavours such as adding lightly sautéed leek and onion, adding mustard or making cheesy mash by mixing in a small handful of cheese.

96

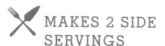

MAKES 2 SIDE SERVINGS

1 Cauliflower head

1 teaspoon butter

Sea salt to taste

Black pepper

Cauli mash

- Steam the cauliflower until soft. If you don't own a steamer, then use a small saucepan with a small volume of water in the bottom. Boil the water, and place the lid on the saucepan and reduce the heat to a simmer. Keep an eye on the volume of water in the saucepan and add a splash or two if the level diminishes

- Once the cauliflower is cooked through and soft, puree using a hand blender

- Leave the cauliflower puree to one side to cool

- Add the butter and seasonings and puree again

- Stir in any optional toppings or ingredients before serving immediately, whilst still hot

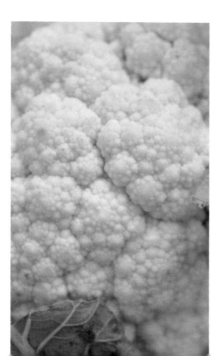

Sweet potato returns again to make a sweeter flavourful mash.

Sweet mash

- Peel the sweet potato and chop into small chunks

- Add these to a sauce pan with enough water to cover the chunks

- Bring to the boil and the reduce to a simmer until the cubes are soft enough to pierce easily with a knife

- Once cooked through, drain the water away

- Add the salt, pepper and butter

- For a smooth mash, puree with a hand blender or for a chunkier texture, mash with a potato masher or fork

- Spoon the mash into a dish and serve as a side

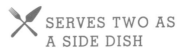

SERVES TWO AS
A SIDE DISH

1 large sweet potato
(approximately 350g)

Coarse sea salt

Black pepper

1 teaspoon butter (optional)

97

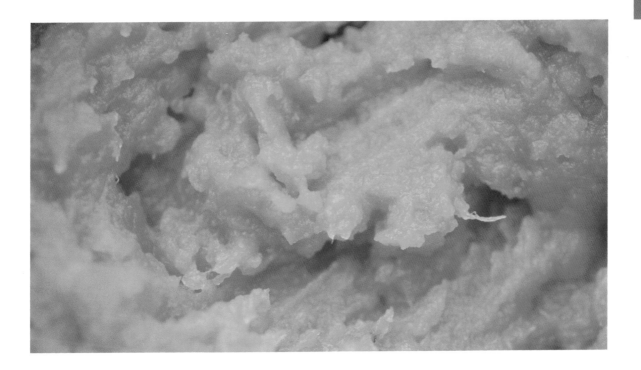

This fresh, sharp coleslaw is unlike the more common creamy, salad cream infused variety. The sweet apples and carrots contrast nicely with the sharpness of the lemon juice, gherkins and vinegar.

Coleslaw

- Wash all vegetables and fruit
- Take the whole cabbages and chop across horizontally, to create thin ribbons of cabbage
- Grate the carrots
- Finely chop the apples, gherkins and peeled spring onion
- Add all ingredients to a large salad bowl and mix together
- Add the vinegar, lemon juice, sea salt and black pepper and mix well
- Serve

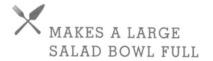

MAKES A LARGE SALAD BOWL FULL

¼ large red cabbage

¼ large white cabbage

4 gherkins

2 apples

2 carrots

1 spring onion

2 tablespoons white wine vinegar

4 tablespoons lemon juice

½ teaspoon coarse sea salt

Black pepper

98

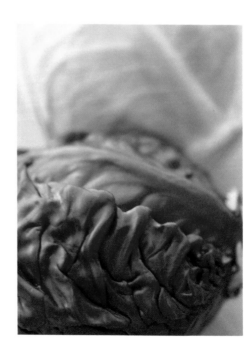

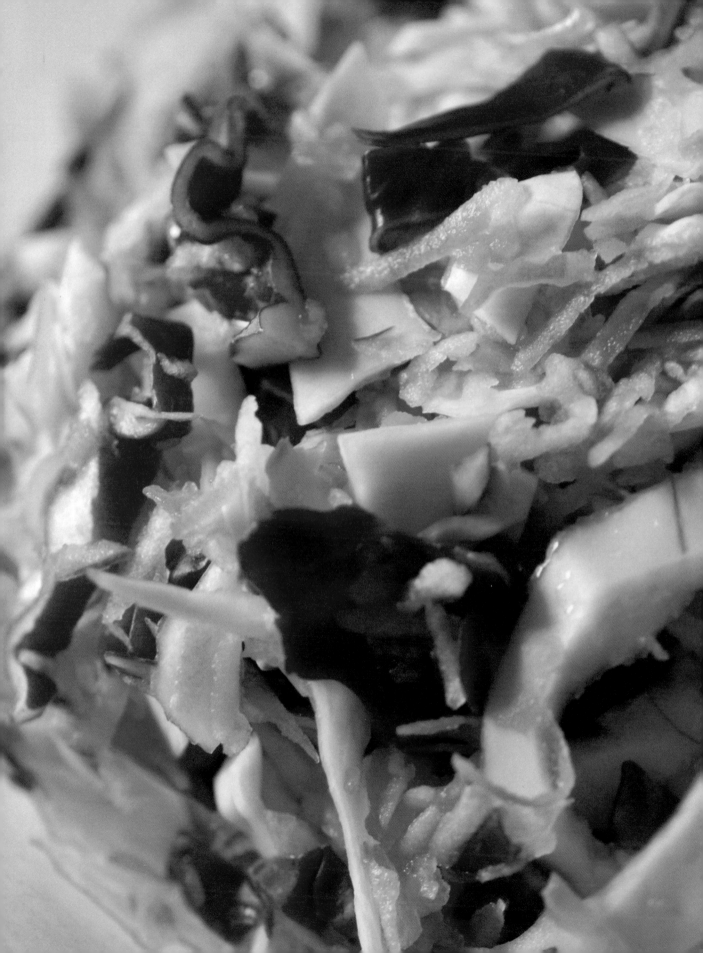

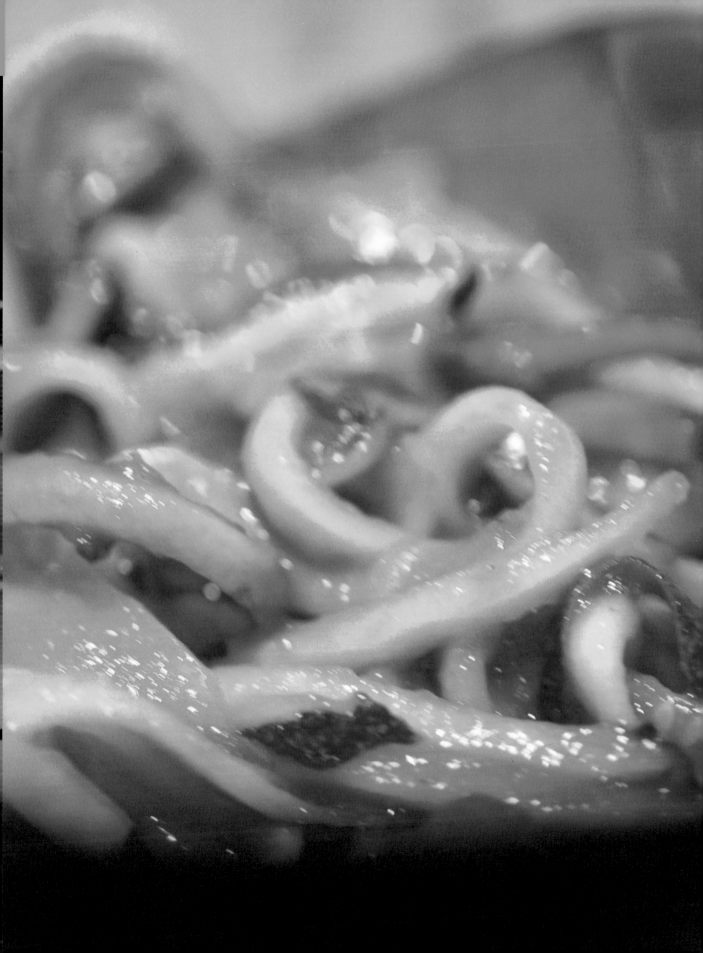

I'm not going to pretend these are the identical clones of grain spaghetti or noodles. However these are delicious in their own right. Beautiful with a generous dollop of pesto mixed in or with my tomato sauce poured over the top, bursting with flavour they far exceed bland beige noodles – no question.

Courgette noodles

- Peel the onion and chop into thin strips

- Sautee in a frying pan on a low heat

- Using a handheld julienne slicer, slice the courgettes lengthways into long thin noodle like strips

- Once the onion starts to show some colour, add the courgette noodles in and turn to a medium heat

- Whilst cooking, add a splash of lemon juice, a small pinch of white pepper and sea salt to taste

- The courgette will turn slightly translucent when cooked through, remove from the heat and either stir in any sauces or additional toppings or serve plain

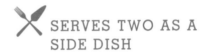

SERVES TWO AS A SIDE DISH

2 courgettes

1 onion

Splash of lemon juice

Large pinch of coarse sea salt

Small pinch of white pepper

1 tablespoon olive oil

101

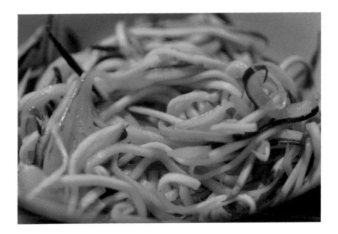

Soft, chunky chips with a uniquely addictive taste.

Colourful chips

- Preheat the oven to 200 degrees celsius (fan assisted oven)

- Peel the sweet potato

- Chop the peeled sweet potato in half and then slice each half into thick rectangular strips

- Spread out the sweet potato chips over a foil lined baking sheet

- Drizzle a generous few glugs of olive oil, enough to coat the chips

- Sprinkle the salt over the chips and mix to evenly coat

- Place in the oven for approximately 20-40 minutes (depending on the thickness of your chips) or until chips are soft enough to pierce with a knife and the edges are starting to turn brown

- Once cooked, remove from the oven and leave to cool slightly before serving warm

SERVES 1-2

1 large sweet potato

Olive oil

Sea salt

102

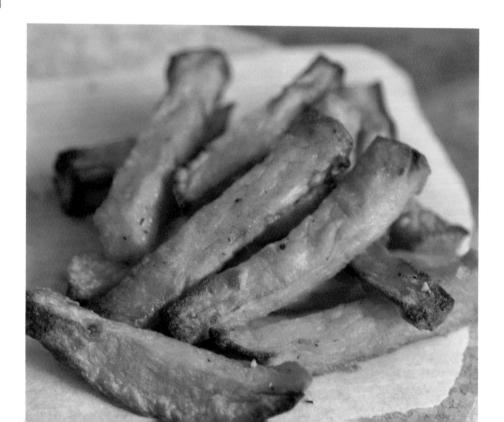

These little green mange tout pods are highly addictive. So healthy, these are my new snacking food. Salty and slightly crunchy perfect for when those crisp cravings hit.

Addictive mange tout

- In a frying pan, heat the olive oil on medium to high

- Once heated, add the mange tout to the pan

- Stir at regular intervals

- When the pods start to turn a brighter shade of green, add the salt, tasting as you go, a few pinches is usually perfect and you can always add more afterward if you find it's not salty enough

- Once there is a hint of brown, remove from the heat and serve in a small dish either as a side dish or just for picking at

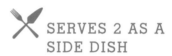 SERVES 2 AS A
SIDE DISH

2 handfuls mange tout

Generous splash olive oil

Sea salt to taste

103

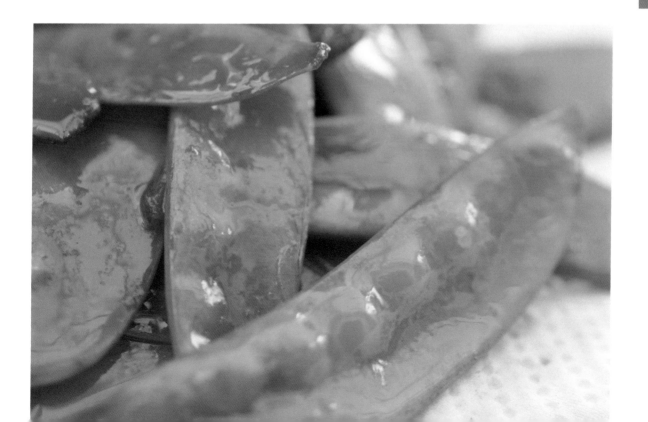

Spicy wedges

- Preheat the oven to 200 degrees celsius (fan assisted oven)

- Peel the sweet potato and chop into chunky wedges

- Spread out the wedges on a greaseproof paper lined baking tray

- Drizzle a generous amount of oil and sprinkle the seasonings over the wedges and toss the wedges to ensure an even covering of oil and spices

- Place in the oven for approximately 40 minutes, turning the wedges occasionally

- Once soft enough to easily pierce with a knife, remove from the oven and leave to cool slightly before eating

✗ SERVES 1-2

1 large sweet potato

Olive oil

⅛ teaspoon cumin

⅛ teaspoon paprika

½ teaspoon oregano

¼ teaspoon sea salt

Black pepper

104

Want a bit more flavour to your chips? Try these sweet yet spicy wedges for a subtle yet flavour filled kick.

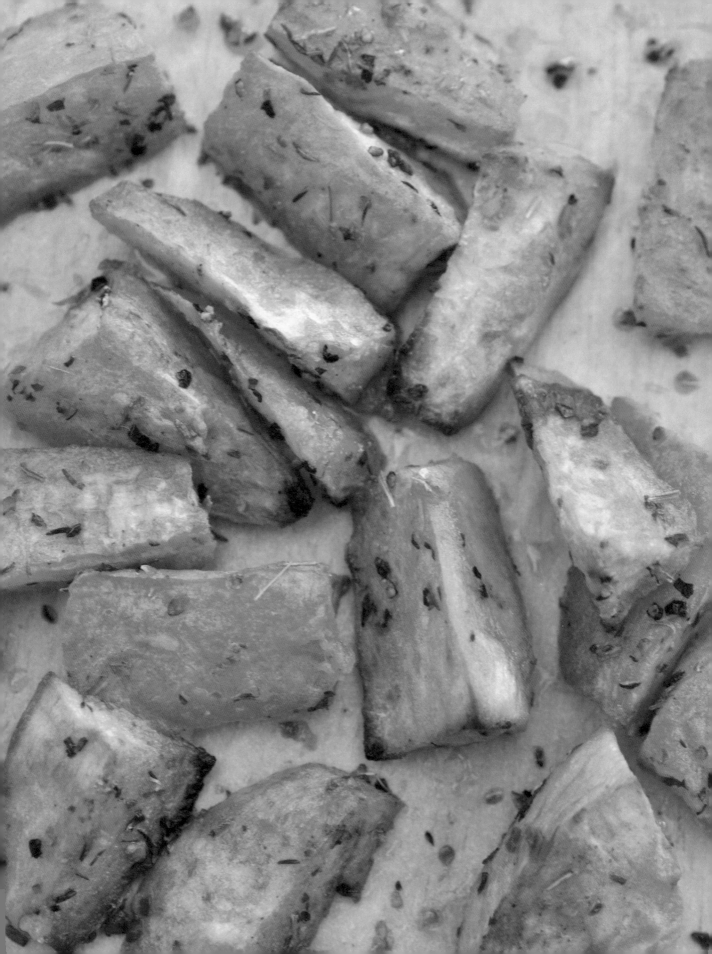

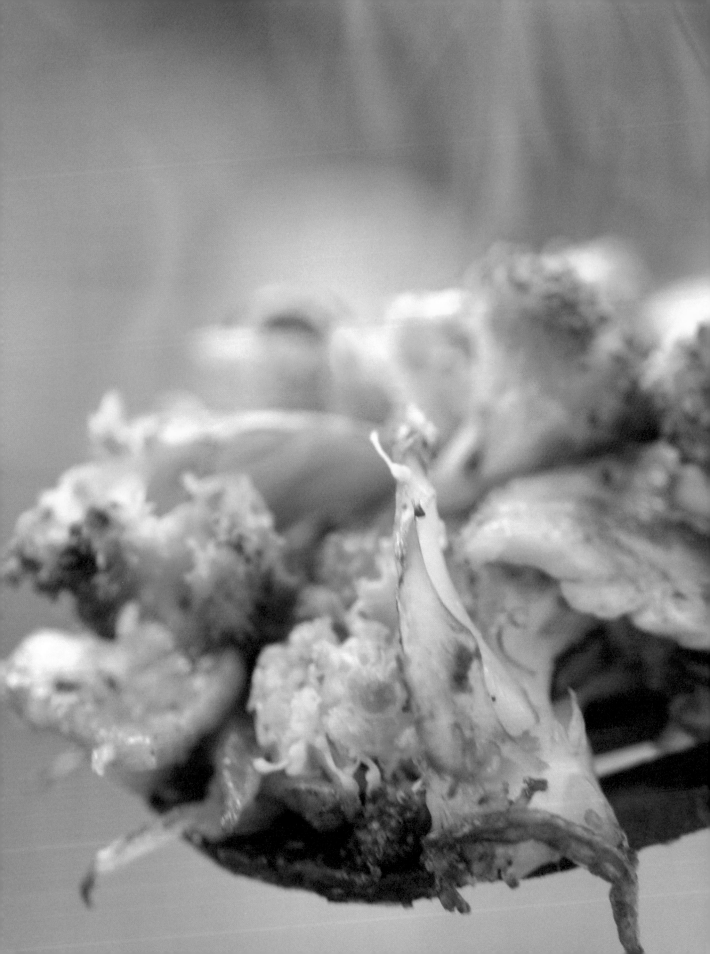

Broccoli, bacon, onion smash

- Break or roughly chop the broccoli into florets

- Steam the broccoli until soft; Do this by heating a centimetre of water in the bottom of the saucepan until it boils. Then place the lid on the saucepan and turn the heat down to a simmer. When the broccoli is soft enough to be easily pierced with a knife, the broccoli is cooked through

- Fry the bacon in a frying pan on medium heat

- Once crispy, remove the bacon from the pan and set aside

- Turn the heat down and add a splash of oil to the frying pan

- Finely chop the onion and add to the frying pan

- Once the onion softens and starts to show a bit of colour, add in the broccoli florets

- Chop the bacon into small pieces and add to the pan

- Continue to fry the mixture, adding in salt and black pepper to taste

- Stir occasionally to evenly cook

- After about 5 minutes, remove from the pan and serve

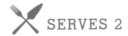 SERVES 2

1 broccoli head

2 onions

Salt

Black pepper

3 rashers bacon

Hazelnut oil

107

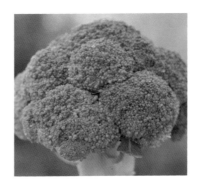

Whenever my Babcia (grandmother) comes to visit we can always rest assured there will be at least one pot of this fresh tomato and kielbasa sitting on the counter before her stay is through.

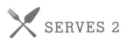 SERVES 2

108

One third of a kielbasa ring

1 large onion

8 large tomatoes

Sea salt to taste

Pinch of white pepper

Kielbasa and tomato

- Bring water to the boil in a saucepan and remove from the heat

- Cut a cross in the top of each tomato to make it easier to peel later

- Place the tomatoes in the hot water and leave to soften for 5 minutes

- Whilst the tomatoes are softening, finely chop the onion and fry in a splash of oil on a low heat until soft

- Take a tomato and using the cross in the top of the tomato, take a corner and peel away the skin. Repeat for the rest of the tomatoes

- Chop the kielbasa into small chunks and add to the fried onions to warm

- Chop the peeled tomatoes, removing the seeds and add the flesh into the pan

- Cover the pan and allow to simmer for 20 minutes, checking the mixture does not dry out and adding a tablespoon or two water if necessary

- Once the tomatoes are soft and warmed through add the salt and white pepper to taste and serve

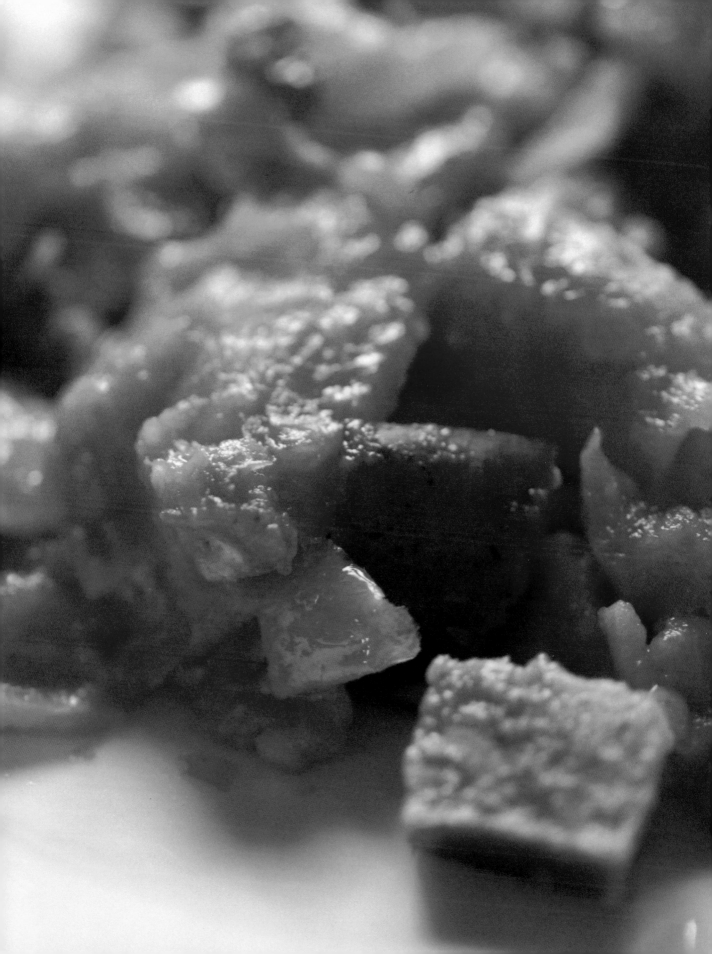

ADDING FLAVOUR AND MOISTURE TO A DISH, SAUCES PROVIDE A SIMPLE BACK GROUND FLAVOUR SUCH AS A DRIZZLE OF OIL OVER A SIMPLE SALAD OR A THICK FLAVOURFUL SAUCE CAN MAKE A POWERFUL ADDITION TO A DISH. OTHER SAUCES ARE ICONIC, WITH A DISTINCTIVE FLAVOUR AND TEXTURE, POPPING UP ON KITCHEN AND RESTAURANT TABLES WORLDWIDE. HOWEVER A LOT OF THESE SMALL CONDIMENTS CONTAIN HEAPS OF HIDDEN SUGARS, FLOURS AND CHEMICAL ADDITIVES. CONCOCTING YOUR OWN SAUCES FREES YOU TO USE THE AMOUNT OF SWEETNESS AND INGREDIENTS YOU CHOOSE, SO YOU CAN CATER SPECIFICALLY TO YOUR TASTES

mmm....saucy

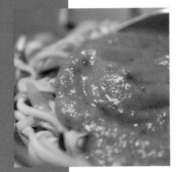

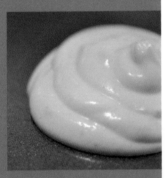

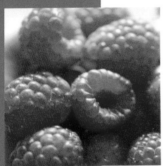

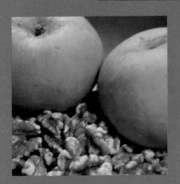

111

6 This versatile tomato sauce can be used as a dip, a pizza sauce or on top of vegetables such as courgette noodles. 9

Tomato sauce

MAKES 300ML

1 small onion

300ml passata

¼ teaspoon oregano

½ teaspoon herbes de provence

Large pinch coarse sea salt

Pinch white pepper

1 tablespoon olive oil

- Peel and finely chop the onion

- Add the onion to a pan with the olive oil and sauté on a low heat

- Once the onion has turned translucent and is starting to show a bit of colour, add the salt, white pepper, oregano and herbes de provence

- Continue to sauté for another minute or two before stirring in the passata

- Bring the sauce to a simmer on a low heat and stir occasionally to let the flavours infuse

- Once heated through, remove from the heat and use a hand blender to blend the sauce until smooth

- Remove the sauce from the pan and use immediately or leave to cool before pouring into a sealable jar and storing in the fridge

112

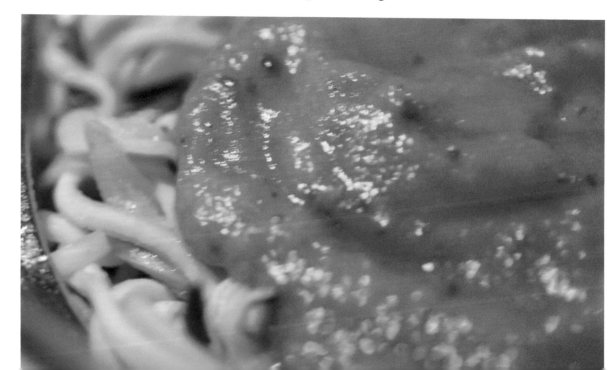

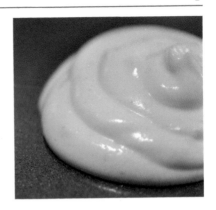

> *The same satay sauce as used in my chicken satay, this sauce can be equally good over salads, veg or other meats.*

Satay sauce

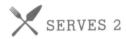 SERVES 2

¼ teaspoon mild chilli powder

¼ teaspoon ginger

⅛ teaspoon cumin

Coarse sea salt to taste

25g coconut

100ml water

4 tablespoons chunky peanut butter

1 teaspoon balsamic vinegar

1 spring onion

- Melt the coconut block in the saucepan with the water on a low heat
- Once the coconut has melted add the peanut butter, mild chilli powder, ginger, cumin and balsamic vinegar and stir
- Add salt to taste
- Serve

Mayonnaise

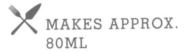 MAKES APPROX. 80ML

3 tablespoons crème fraiche

50ml walnut oil

Black pepper

Pinch paprika

Sea salt to taste

¼ teaspoon mustard

1 teaspoon lemon juice

- Mix together the crème fraiche, pepper, paprika, mustard and lemon juice
- Slowly add the walnut oil whilst stirring
- Add salt to taste
- Use immediately or store in a sealed container in the fridge

> *I may be alone in this but I feel a little uneasy eating raw egg. Three tablespoons of crème fraiche, take the place of the egg yolks in this fresh mayonnaise.*

113

Tomato ketchup from scratch gives you control over the amount of sweetness you put in.

Serve on the side of meat dishes and adjust the amount of honey used to your taste.

Ketchup

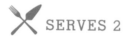 SERVES 2

100ml tomato passata

1 teaspoon tomato puree

¼ teaspoon ground mixed spice

1 teaspoon white wine vinegar

¼ teaspoon coarse sea salt

1 teaspoon honey

Pinch white pepper

- Add all the ingredients to a small saucepan on a low to medium heat

- Stir the mixture and reduce until it thickens to the desired thickness

- Remove from the heat and allow to cool

- Serve immediately or store in a sealed container in the fridge

Apple sauce

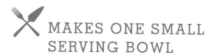 MAKES ONE SMALL SERVING BOWL

1 cooking apple

1 teaspoon lemon juice

Pinch cinnamon

Pinch salt

Honey to taste

- Peel and chop the cooking apple and stew the apple pieces in a saucepan with a splash of water on a low heat

- Cook on a low heat until the apple pieces become soft and break down, creating a thick sauce

- Add the lemon juice, cinnamon, salt and honey to taste

- Once cooked through, remove from the heat and serve immediately or allow to cool before storing

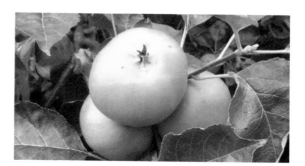

114

Gravy from a stock cube usually has a strong flavour and an addictive quality. This isn't highly surprising with the amount of additives, MSG, sugar etc. To make this simple gravy, use my fresh stock described earlier or you can find some liquid stocks available which contain no extra nasties.

Gravy

- Melt the butter in a small saucepan on a low heat

- Finely chop the shallots and add to the saucepan to sauté

- Once the onions have turned transparent and are starting to show a bit of colour, add the pepper, thyme and balsamic vinegar and stir

- Add the stock and tomato puree

- Bring to the boil for 2-3 minutes and then reduce to a simmer for approximately 10 minutes, adding coconut flour gradually to thicken until the desired consistency is reached

- Add salt to taste

- Always add in any extra juices left over from roasting meats to give more flavour

- Serve hot in a gravy boat or pour directly over your dish

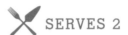 SERVES 2

2 shallots

1 teaspoon butter

1 teaspoon balsamic vinegar

300ml stock

¼ teaspoon coarse sea salt

Pinch white pepper

½ teaspoon thyme

1 teaspoon tomato puree

Coconut flour

115

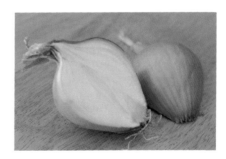

A fruity sauce, great as a side with duck.

Raspberry, mango sauce

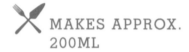 MAKES APPROX. 200ML

100g raspberries

½ mango

160ml water

1 teaspoon balsamic vinegar

- Add the raspberries and half the water to a sauce pan on a low to medium heat
- Stew the raspberries until they breakdown
- Pass the raspberry mixture through a sieve to sieve out the pips and return the pip-free sauce to the saucepan
- Add the rest of the water and the chopped mango to the saucepan
- Keep the mixture simmering on a low to medium heat, stirring occasionally
- Once the mango is fairly soft, use a hand blender to puree the sauce until smooth
- Keep simmering on a low heat until the sauce reaches a viscous consistency
- Once the desired thickness is reached, remove the sauce from the heat and either serve warm over a warm dish or pour into a bowl and allow to cool before serving over a cold dish

Balsamic and hazelnut vinaigrette

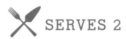 SERVES 2

30ml balsamic vinegar

30ml hazelnut oil

15ml lemon juice

Coarse sea salt to taste

- Pour the balsamic vinegar and lemon juice in a small bowl
- Whilst stirring constantly, slowly pour in the hazelnut oil
- Once the oil has been mixed in, the vinaigrette will become thicker, now you can add the salt to taste
- Serve over leaves or salads

A great addition to sweet fruity salads, such as my strawberry salad.

❝ Smooth, thick dressing, using a whole apple instead of highly sugary concentrated apple juice; this makes a thick, naturally sweet salad sauce. ❞

❝ As an exceedingly sweet syrup, you only need to use a small amount to give a citrus kick. ❞

Apple and walnut dressing

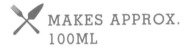 MAKES APPROX. 100ML

1 teaspoon lemon juice

1 eating apple

30ml water

30ml walnut oil

Large pinch coarse sea salt

- Peel, deseed and chop an eating apple

- Puree the apple, sea salt, water and walnut oil in a high speed blender until it reaches a smooth consistency

- Pour over salad or leaves

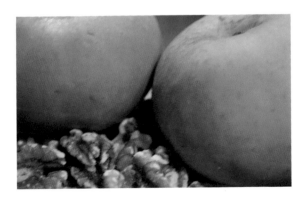

Sweet lemon honey syrup

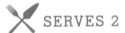 SERVES 2

2 tablespoons honey

50ml lemon juice

- Add the honey to a saucepan over medium heat

- Stir the honey as it starts to bubble and froth until it starts to turn a deeper shade of brown, continuously stir the honey and keep a close eye on the temperature as you don't want the honey to burn

- Once a deeper shade, turn the temperature down to a low heat and add the lemon juice

- To reduce the syrup, keep stirring, whilst simmering on a low heat for about 5 minutes

- Take the saucepan off the heat and leave to cool

- When ready, drizzle the syrup over muffins, salads or pancakes

117

ICINGS AND TOPPINGS ARE TREATS, USUALLY TOOTH ACHINGLY SWEET; THEY ARE USED TO GIVE A DISH AN EXTRA SPECIAL SOMETHING. WITH LIMITED HONEY AND SWEET ELEMENTS IN THESE TOPPINGS, A LITTLE GOES A LONG WAY. SO NOW YOU CAN GIVE A SCRUMPTIOUS KICK TO YOUR FAVOURITE DESSERTS!

tasty toppings

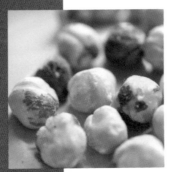

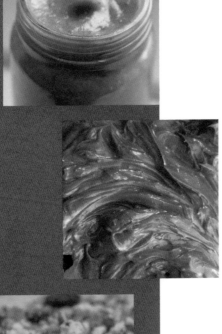

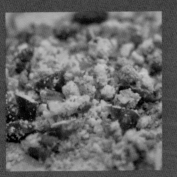

119

A brilliant topping plain and simple or with a drizzle of honey for an added sweetness, pipe on top of cakes for a swirled topping.

Whipped cream

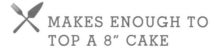 **MAKES ENOUGH TO TOP A 8″ CAKE**

200ml cream

Few drops vanilla essence (optional)

Drizzle of honey (optional)

- Pour the cream into a bowl
- Use an electric whisk to whip the cream
- Once the cream has reached soft peaks add a drizzle of honey and the vanilla essence and whisk further
- Spread or pipe on top of cakes or add a spoonful to a slice of pie or a handful of fresh berries

120

Honey vanilla icing

MAKES ENOUGH TO TOP ONE CARROT CAKE (SEE SINLESS SWEETS)

50ml double cream

100g cream cheese

1 teaspoon vanilla extract

1½ tablespoons honey

Pinch salt

- Using an electric whisk, whisk the double cream till stiff peaks form
- Add the cream cheese, vanilla extract, honey and salt and whisk until you're left with smooth and creamy icing
- Keep the icing covered in the fridge until ready to use

This icing makes a wonderful staple icing for anything from carrot cake to individual cupcakes.

Candied hazelnuts

Sprinkle over the top of salads or crème fraiche and fruit to give a nutty crunch.

- Preheat the oven to 150 degrees celsius (fan assisted)

- Line a baking tray with greaseproof paper

- Mix together the hazelnuts, hazelnut oil, honey and salt and spread out over the baking sheet

- Place in the oven for approximately 10-15 minutes, turning the hazelnuts every 5 minutes to roast the hazelnuts evenly

- Once slightly brown around the edges, remove the hazelnuts from the oven and leave to cool for approximately 10 minutes

- Once cooled, store in a sealed container or sealable plastic bag

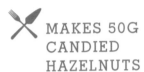

MAKES 50G
CANDIED
HAZELNUTS

50g hazelnuts

1 teaspoon honey

1½ tablespoon hazelnut oil

Pinch salt

121

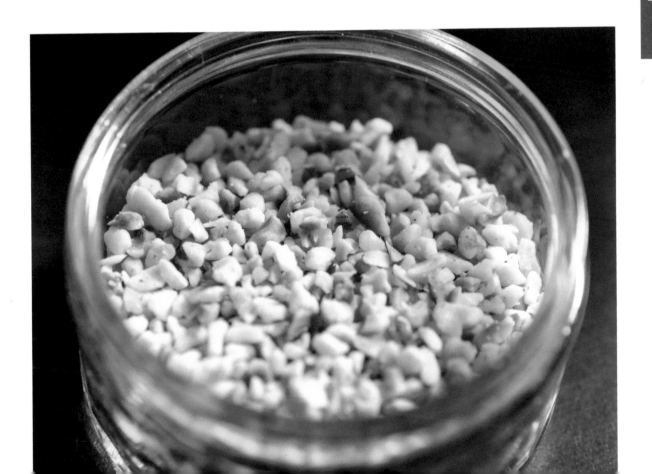

Oooooh caramel… truly sinful! Consisting mostly of sugar, this sauce is usually a strict no- no when lowering sugar content. However, searching for a natural caramel didn't turn out to be too difficult. Pureed dates can make a thick creamy spreadable caramel for topping cakes or fillings.

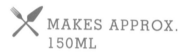

MAKES APPROX.
150ML

100g dates

100ml water

1 tablespoon butter

50ml double cream

Perfectly spreadable, I use this caramel in recipes such as millionaire shortbread and banoffee pie.

122

Thick caramel

- Add the dates and water to a saucepan on low heat and allow to simmer until the dates start to soften

- Once the dates are soft and the water begins to become absorbed by the dates, add the butter and cream

- Mix in the ingredients and once the dates are soft enough and the butter has just melted, use a hand blender to blend the date mixture into a smooth, thick puree

- Allow the date puree to cool before using or spooning into a jar and storing in the fridge

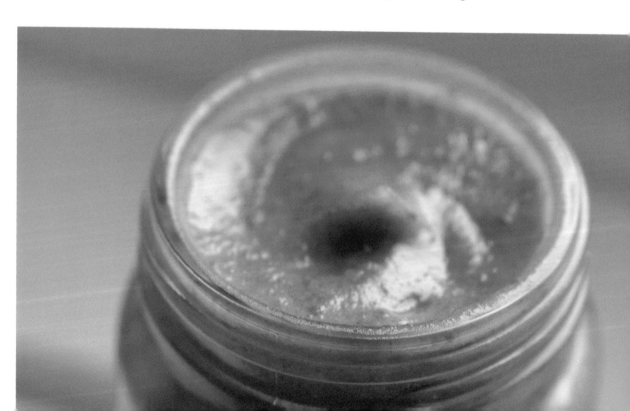

The second caramel sauce is better for swirling into a milkshake for a sweet kick. Definitely a worthwhile swap for ordinary caramel sauces.

Caramel sauce

- Place the honey in a small saucepan on a low heat

- As the honey heats it will become less sticky and more runny

- As you stir the honey, it should start to bubble, let it bubble for 2 minutes or until it turns a slightly deeper shade of golden brown

- At this stage, add the cashew butter and vanilla essence, stirring into the honey

- Add the cream and stir together, keeping on a low heat until the desired consistency has been reached

- Remove the caramel from the heat and leave to cool before pouring into a sealable jar to store in the fridge

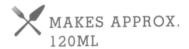 MAKES APPROX. 120ML

3 tablespoons honey

1 tablespoon cashew butter

100ml cream

½ teaspoon vanilla essence

123

Drizzle over ice cream or into milkshakes. A little goes a long way!

❛Gorgeously thick custard. Pour whilst still hot over a slice of Christmas cake or mince pie.❜

Custard

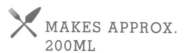

MAKES APPROX. 200ML

1½ tablespoon honey

120ml milk

1 tablespoon vanilla essence

1½ tablespoons cashew butter

100ml cream

Pinch salt

- Place the honey in a small saucepan on a low heat

- The honey will start to become less sticky and more runny as you stir it

- The honey will then start to bubble and froth. Watch for a colour change, and after a minute or two the honey will turn a slightly deeper golden brown colour

- Add the cashew butter, salt and vanilla essence and stir together

- Add the milk and heat until just about to start boiling, then turn the heat down and simmer on a low heat

- Add the cream and mix together

- Keep stirring the mixture over a low heat until the desired consistency is reached and the mixture has heated through

- Once the mixture has reached a thick consistency, remove from the heat and either serve immediately for warm custard or allow to cool before serving cold

124

I use this simple butter icing in my Victoria sponge cake. Always make this icing fresh, just before you intend to use it.

A variation on the simple butter icing, this chocolate butter icing brings back memories of childhood birthday cakes but without the sugar rush!

Butter icing

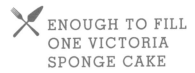 ENOUGH TO FILL
ONE VICTORIA
SPONGE CAKE

75g butter

50ml double cream

1 tablespoon honey

- Add the room temperature butter to a small bowl

- Using an electric whisk, start to cream the butter

- Whilst whisking, slowly pour in the cream (cold from the fridge)

- Finally add the honey and continue to whisk until a creamy, silky mixture has been reached

- Spread on a completely cooled cake

Chocolate butter icing

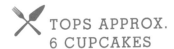 TOPS APPROX.
6 CUPCAKES

50g butter

1 tablespoon cocoa powder

1½ tablespoon honey

- Using a whisk, cream the room temperature butter together with the cocoa and honey

- Use immediately, spreading on completely cooled cakes

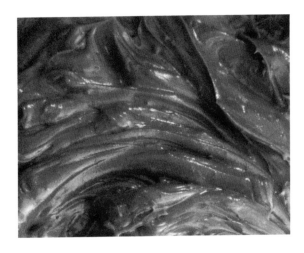

125

> *I make a large amount of this pecan topping and keep in a sealed jar until I feel the need for my breakfast bowl (see blissful bowls).*

Crumbly pecan topping

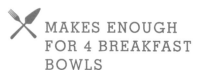

MAKES ENOUGH FOR 4 BREAKFAST BOWLS

Handful pecans

100g ground almonds

50g flaked almonds

2 tablespoons honey

1 tablespoon butter

Large pinch cinnamon

Splash vanilla essence

6 chopped dates

- Preheat the oven to 150 degrees celsius (fan assisted oven)

- Roughly chop the pecans and add to a mixing bowl along with the ground almonds, flaked almonds and cinnamon

- Add room temperature butter, honey and vanilla essence into the bowl and mix together using a crumbling action with your hands - picking up handfuls of mixture and crumbling it between your fingers, sprinkling it back into the bowl

- Line a baking tray with greaseproof paper and spread out the mixture

- Bake for 10 – 15 minutes, turning the mixture over every few minutes to bake evenly

- Once baked and golden brown, remove from the oven and leave to cool

- Once fully cooled, finely chop the dates and add to the mixture

- Keep in a sealable container to keep fresh

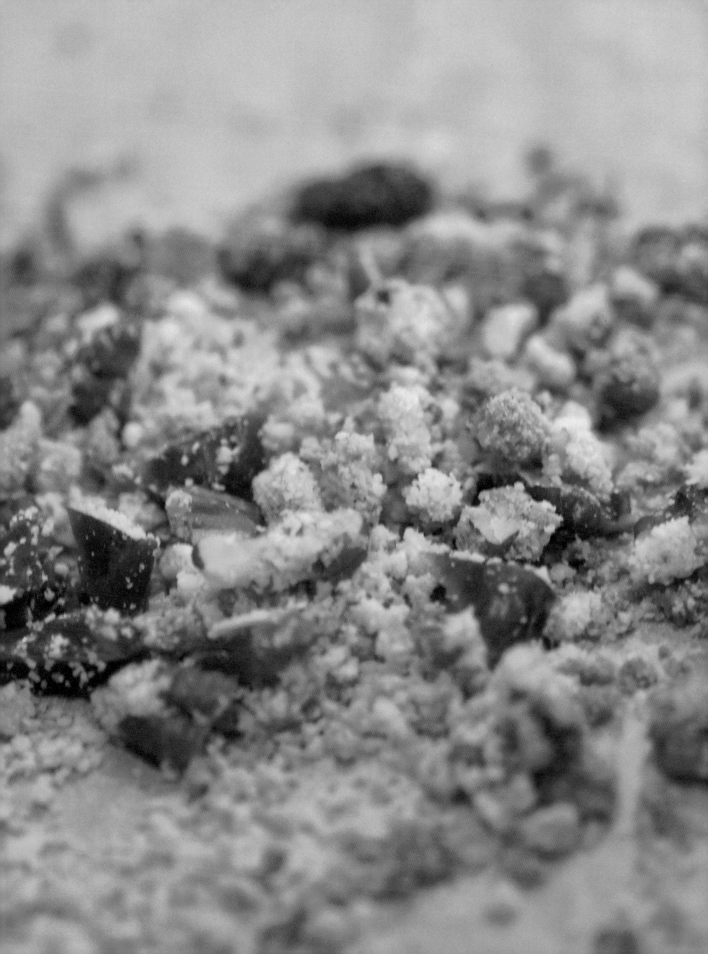

SWEETS AND DESSERTS WITH THEIR
UNBELIEVABLY HIGH SUGAR AND GRAIN
CONTENT ARE USUALLY THE FIRST TO GO IN
THE QUEST FOR OPTIMAL HEALTH. CAUSING
THIS GENRE OF FOOD TO BE THE MOST
SORELY MISSED. THE WIDELY AVAILABLE
HIGHLY PROCESSED SUGARY TREATS SEEM
TO POP UP EVERYWHERE. CONSTANTLY
TEMPTING, ALMOST TAUNTING… SO THIS
SECTION IS SPECIFICALLY FOR THOSE
TIMES WHEN A SLICE OF NOSTALGIA AND
COMFORT IS NEEDED BUT WITHOUT THE
HEALTH COSTS. CREATING CAKES AND
SWEET BITES WITH NUTS, FRUITS AND
SMALL AMOUNTS OF SWEETER FOODS
MAKES FOR A SINLESS INDULGENCE

sinless sweets

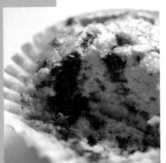

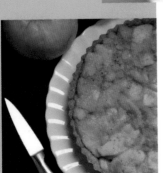

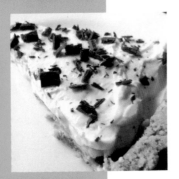

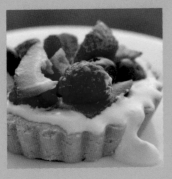

129

Rustic carrot cake

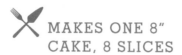

MAKES ONE 8″ CAKE, 8 SLICES

125g carrot

1 egg white

½ lemon zest

Pinch salt

50g coconut butter

1 tablespoon honey

100g ground almonds

Handful pecans

50g dates

¼ teaspoon bicarbonate of soda

¼ teaspoon cinnamon

Pinch ginger

⅛ teaspoon ground mixed spice

1 Honey vanilla icing recipe (see tasty toppings)

- Preheat the oven to 160 degrees celsius (fan assisted oven)

- Grate the carrots and add into a mixing bowl along with the egg white, lemon zest, salt, coconut butter, honey, ground almonds, bicarbonate of soda, cinnamon, ginger and ground mixed spices

- Chop the pecans and dates and add to the bowl and mix in

- Line an 8 inch circular baking tin with greaseproof paper

- Pour the mixture into the tin and place in the oven to bake for approximately 30 minutes

- Whilst the cake is cooking, make the icing and keep refrigerated until needed

- Once the cake is done, it will turn golden brown on top and become firmer, test whether the cake is done by sticking a knife through the centre of the cake, if the knife comes out clean the cake is done

- Remove the cake from the oven and leave to cool

- Once cooled, use a knife to frost the top of the cake with the icing you made earlier

- Decorate with a few walnuts, coconut flakes, desiccated coconut or if trying to impress then carve a small carrot from the tip of a carrot. For the green leaf, take a leaf of spinach and cut the leaf into the shape of a club or carrot top, placing it behind the carrot on the top of the cake

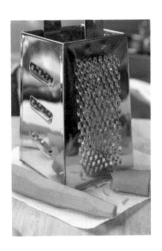

This is such a simply beautiful cake. With a subtle sweetness, this moist cake is bursting with fresh carrot flavour, frosted with a creamy honey vanilla icing. Definitely a must for Easter.

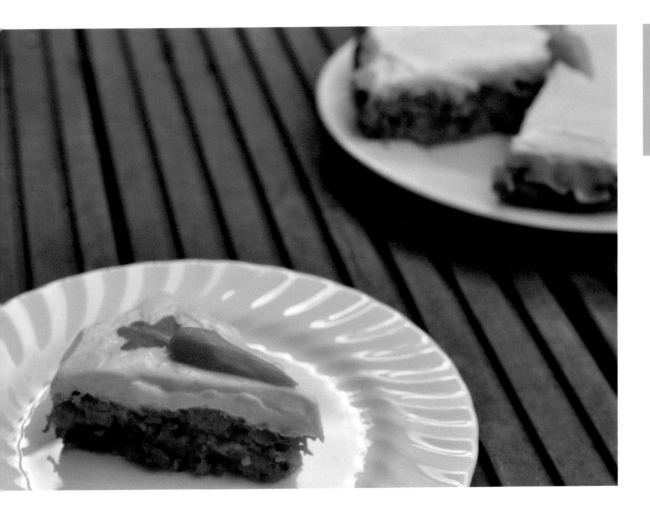

**What can you say about a Victoria sponge? It's THE classic cake, making it perfect for almost any occasion. Like a little black dress, this cake can be dressed up for a birthday party or special occasion or dressed down for a normal everyday pick me up.**

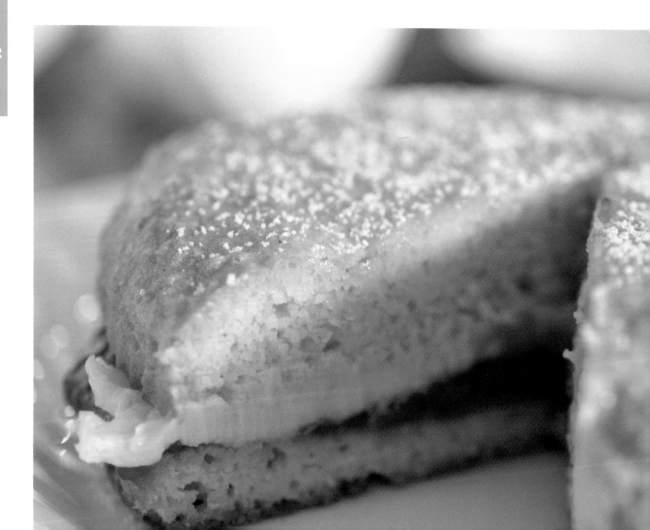

A very English Victoria sponge

- Preheat the oven to 160 degrees celsius (fan assisted oven)

- Add the ground almonds, melted butter, honey, bicarbonate of soda and vanilla essence into a bowl

- In a second bowl, use an electric whisk to whip the egg whites into stiff peaks

- Add one quarter of the whipped egg whites to the first bowl and using a spoon, cut the egg whites into the mixture. Be careful not to over mix, as you want to keep as much air in the mixture as possible, as this gives the cake its height

- Continue to add the egg whites a quarter at a time until all the egg whites are incorporated into the mixture

- Line a round 8" cake tin with a circular greaseproof liner

- Pour the mixture into the tin and carefully spread out until the mixture is even

- Place in the oven and bake for 20-30 minutes or until the cake is golden brown on top. When you are able to stick a knife through the centre of the cake with it coming out clean, the cake is done

- Remove the cake from the oven and leave to cool

- Once cooled, cut the cake in half and separate the two circular layers

- On the bottom half of the cake spread some strawberry jam (I use St Dalfour) or cut up and layer some fresh slices of strawberries

- Turn the top half of the cake upside down and spread a thick layer of icing over the surface

- Sandwich the two halves of the cake together

- For an extra finishing touch, you could crush some palm sugar to a fine powder and sprinkle over the top of the cake and you're ready to serve

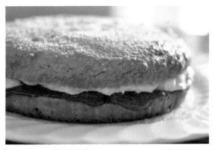

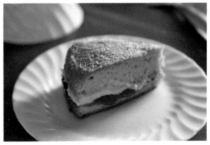

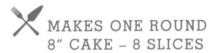

133

MAKES ONE ROUND 8" CAKE – 8 SLICES

200g ground almonds

75g butter

1½ tablespoons honey

½ tsp bicarbonate of soda

½ tsp vanilla

5 egg whites

It just wouldn't be Christmas without Christmas cake. A season infamous for overeating and a last blow out before new years resolutions kick in. Well no more. You can now have your cake and eat it too! So enjoy a guilt free Christmas, cake and all.

MAKES ONE 8" CIRCULAR CAKE, 8 SLICES

200g cooking apple

50g butter

50g dates

50g pecans

25g hazelnuts

25g dried cranberries

50g currants

50g sultanas

50g raisins

½ teaspoon vanilla essence

1 teaspoon ground mixed spice

½ teaspoon cinnamon

Pinch nutmeg

1 lemon zest and juice

1 clementine zest and juice

200g ground almonds

4 egg whites

½ teaspoon bicarbonate soda

2 tablespoons French brandy

3 tablespoons honey

Pinch sea salt

Fruity Christmas cake

- Preheat the oven to 160 degrees celsius (fan assisted oven)

- Peel and chop the cooking apple and measure out 200g

- Heat the chopped apple with the butter in a saucepan on low heat

- Heat until the apple is stewed and remove from the heat

- Add the ground mixed spice, cinnamon, nutmeg, vanilla essence, brandy, honey, salt, finely grated lemon and clementine zest and juice

- Chop the dates, dried cranberries, hazelnuts and pecans into smaller chunks and add to a separate large mixing bowl

- Add the ground almonds, bicarbonate soda, raisins, currants and sultanas to the mixing bowl

- Finally add in the apple mixture and mix together

- In a separate bowl, use an electric whisk to whip the egg whites into stiff peaks

- Add the egg whites a quarter at a time to the cake mixture and with a spoon, cut into the mixture to incorporate the egg whites

- Continue to do this until all the egg whites are used up

- Line an 8" circular baking tin with greaseproof paper

- Pour the cake mixture into the baking tin and bake in the oven for approximately 50 minutes to one hour or until the cake is firm and the top of the cake turns a deeper brown

- Remove the cake from the oven and leave to cool

- Before you are about to serve, use freshly made icing to frost the cake

- Of course, you can achieve crisper, sharper whirls with minimal mess if you have a piping bag with nozzles. However if you find yourself without – fear not! To make whirled icing, cut a square of greaseproof paper fold in half and then half again

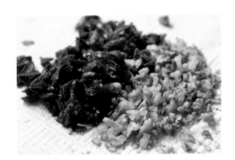

- At the only completely sealed corner, cut off the amount desired. The bigger the corner cut off, the larger the whirls will be

- Spread a thin layer of icing to completely cover the cake

- Pipe whirls all over the cake

135

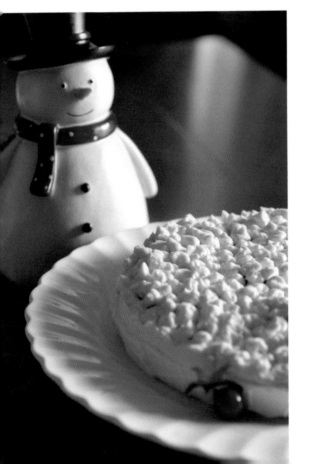

Cream cheese icing

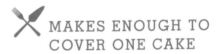 MAKES ENOUGH TO COVER ONE CAKE

400g cream cheese

1½ teaspoon vanilla essence

1 tablespoon lemon juice

2½ tablespoons honey

Make this icing and frost the cake just before serving.

- Use an electric whisk to whip the cream cheese, vanilla essence, lemon juice and honey until it reaches a smooth and creamy consistency

- Store in the fridge until ready to use

Eat plain, cut in half and fill, dress them up with extravagant toppings or add chopped dried fruits and nuts to make every bite interesting. Fill mini cupcakes cases for cute bite size cakes, perfect for parties.

Vanilla cupcakes

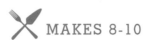 MAKES 8-10

175g ground almonds

4 egg whites

2 tablespoons honey

1 tablespoon vanilla essence

Pinch salt

1 tablespoon lemon juice

½ teaspoon bicarbonate soda

60ml walnut oil

40ml water

- Preheat the oven to 160 degrees celsius (fan assisted oven)

- Add the honey, vanilla essence, salt, lemon juice, bicarbonate of soda, walnut oil, water and ground almonds to a large mixing bowl and mix

- In a second bowl use an electric whisk to whip the egg white to stiff peaks

- Add the egg whites quarter by quarter, cutting them into the cake mixture

- Line a cupcake tray with cupcake cases

- Gently spoon the batter into the cupcake cases until each one is three quarters full

- Place the tray in the oven for approximately 20 minutes or until the cakes turn deeper golden brown

- Once cooked, remove the tray from the oven and leave to cool for about 10 minutes

- Serve as you wish, plain or dressed up!

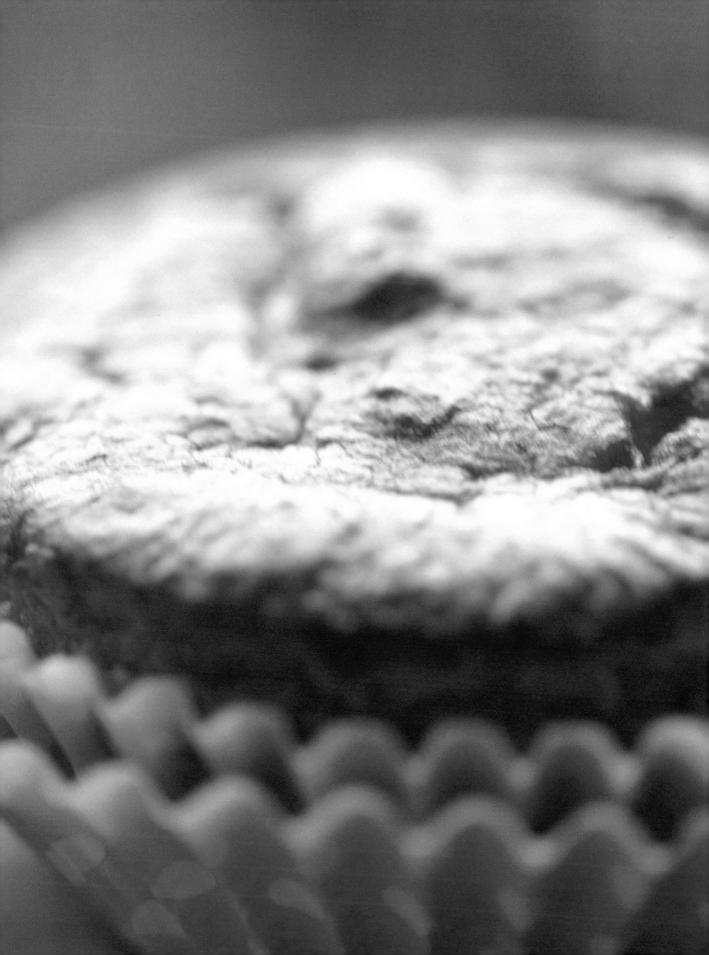

A subtle lemon flavoured muffin, topped with a generous drizzle of sweet lemon honey syrup.

138

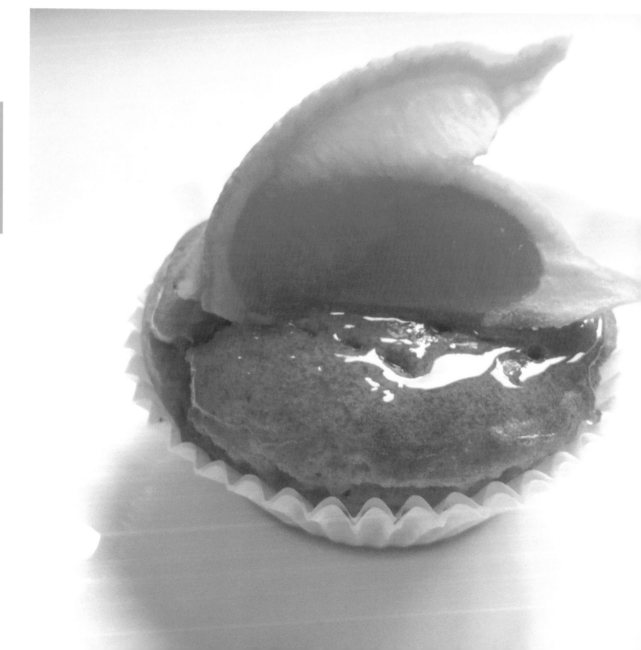

Fresh lemon muffins

- Preheat the oven to 150 degrees celsius (fan assisted oven)

- In a large mixing bowl, add the ground almonds, lemon zest, honey, salt, bicarbonate of soda, water, butter and vanilla essence and mix

- In a second bowl, use an electric whisk to whip the egg whites into stiff peaks

- Add a third of the egg whites to the mixture and use a chopping action with a spoon to incorporate these into the mixture

- Repeat this process until all the egg whites are mixed in

- Line a cupcake tray with cupcake cases

- Gently spoon the mixture into each of the cases until they are three quarters filled and place in the oven for approximately 20 minutes or until turning lightly golden brown

- Remove from the oven and leave to cool

- Make the Lemon honey syrup

- Once cooled, use a fork to poke a few holes in the top of each muffin and then spoon the lemon honey syrup over the top of each muffin to serve

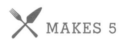 MAKES 5

100g ground almonds

2 egg whites

Zest of one lemon

1 tablespoon honey

Pinch coarse sea salt

¼ teaspoon bicarbonate soda

20ml water

50g butter

1 teaspoon lemon essence

1 Lemon honey syrup recipe (see mmm...saucy)

139

Hazelnutty muffins

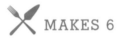 MAKES 6

2 egg whites

1 teaspoon vanilla essence

1 teaspoon lemon juice

2 tablespoons honey

75g hazelnuts

1 tablespoon butter

½ teaspoon bicarbonate soda

25g ground almonds

140

- Preheat the oven to 150 degrees celsius (fan assisted oven)

- Place the hazelnuts in a blender or grinder and pulse until the nuts reach a coarse flour

- Add the ground hazelnuts to a bowl along with the ground almonds, butter, lemon juice, vanilla essence and bicarbonate soda and mix together

- In a separate bowl, whisk the egg whites until they form stiff peaks

- Add a third of the egg whites to the mixture and using a chopping action, mix the egg whites into the mixture. Repeat this process until all the egg whites are used up and incorporated into the mixture

- Gently spoon the mixture into each of the cases until they are three quarters filled and place in the oven for 15-20 minutes or until slightly firm to the touch

- Remove from the oven and leave to cool before serving

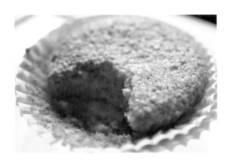

Sweet and nutty, perfect plain or top with my chocolate butter icing.

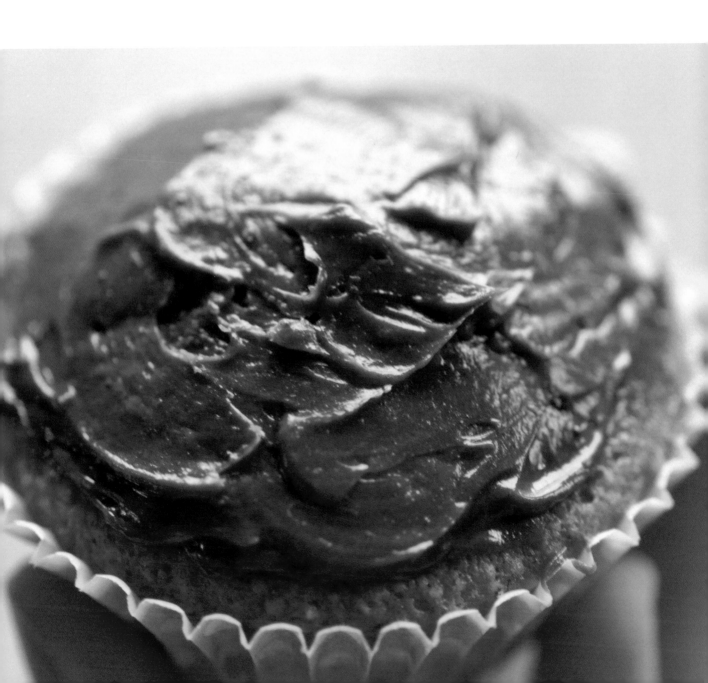

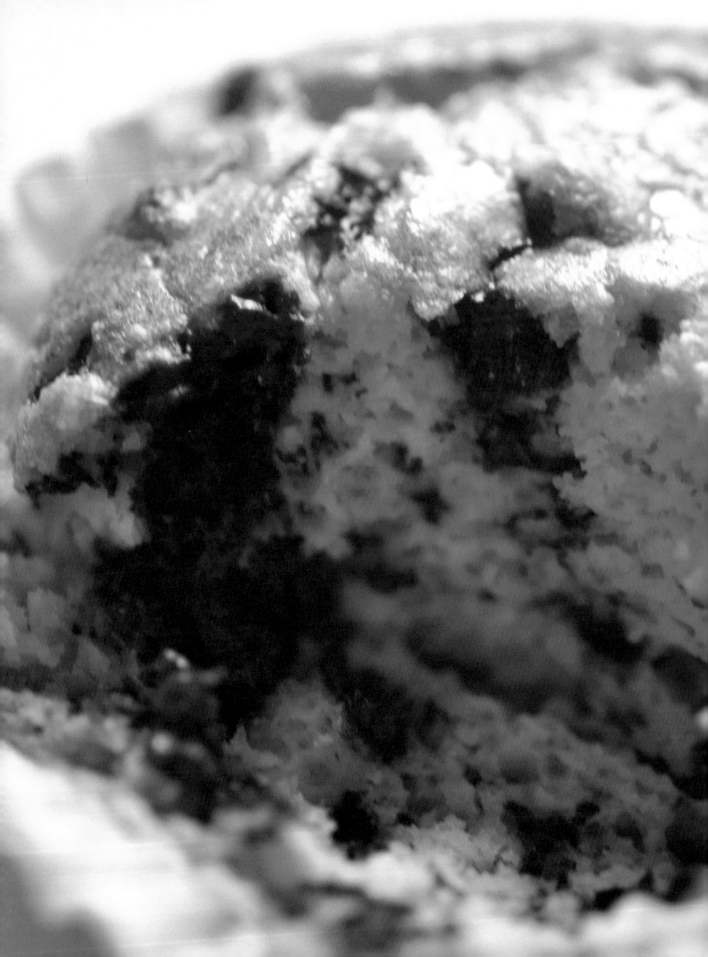

Chocolate chip muffins

- Preheat the oven to 150 degrees celsius (fan assisted oven)

- In a large mixing bowl, add the ground almonds, honey, vanilla essence, bicarbonate of soda, walnut oil, water and salt

- Chop the dark chocolate into small chunks and add to the mixture

- In a second bowl, use an electric whisk to whip the egg whites into stiff peaks

- Add the egg whites quarter by quarter, cutting them into the cake mixture

- Repeat this process until all the egg whites are mixed in

- Line a cupcake tray with cupcake cases

- Gently spoon the mixture into each of the cases until they are three quarters filled and place in the oven for approximately 20 minutes or until turning lightly golden brown

- Remove from the oven and leave to cool

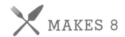 MAKES 8

175g ground almonds

100g 70% dark chocolate

4 egg whites

2 tablespoons honey

2 tablespoon vanilla essence

½ teaspoon bicarbonate soda

60ml walnut oil

40ml water

Pinch coarse sea salt

143

Chocolate chunk loaded. Oh yes.

Have one of these muffins in the place of a granola bar. Packed full of seeds and dried fruits, these crunchy muffins are a perfect on the go snack.

Sophisticated breakfast muffins

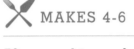 MAKES 4-6

50g pumpkin seeds

2 egg whites

25g walnuts

2 tablespoons water

½ teaspoon bicarbonate soda

25g dried cranberries

25g dried apricots

- Preheat the oven to 160 degrees celsius (fan assisted oven)
- Use a nut/seed grinder or blender to finely grind the pumpkin seeds into a coarse flour and add to a mixing bowl
- Finely chop the walnuts and add to the mixing bowl
- Also add the bicarbonate soda and dried fruit
- In a separate bowl, whisk the egg whites into stiff peaks
- Add a third of the egg whites and delicately use a cutting action to mix into the dry mixture
- Repeat this action until all the egg whites are used
- Line a cupcake tray with cupcake cases and fill the cases with the mixture
- Place in the oven to cook for 15-20 minutes
- Once firm to the touch and cooked through, remove from the oven and leave to cool
- Grab one for breakfast or a quick snack

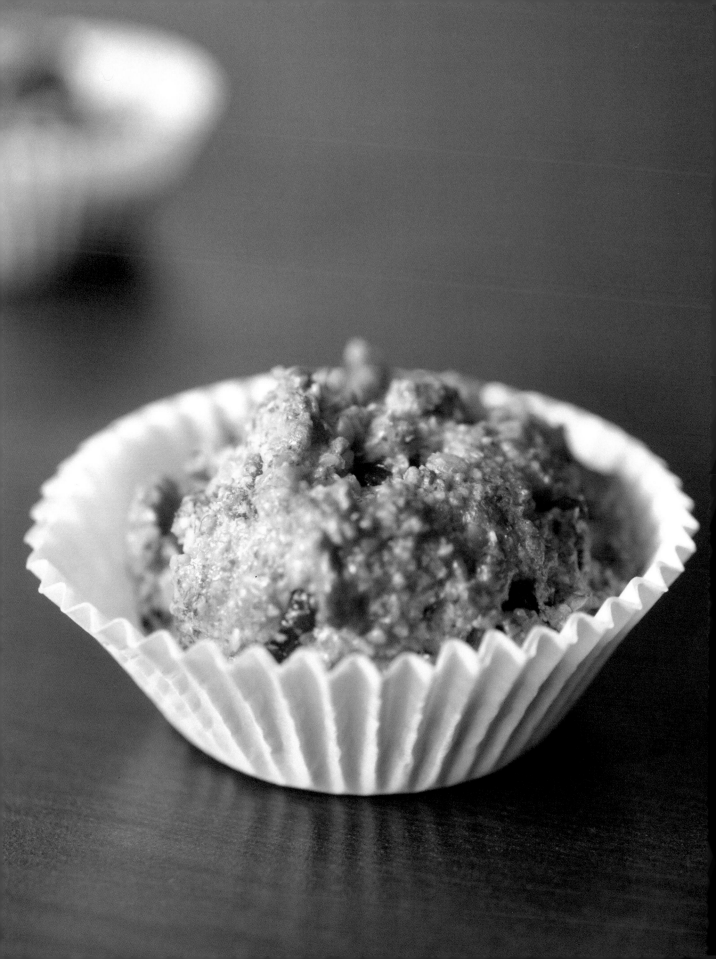

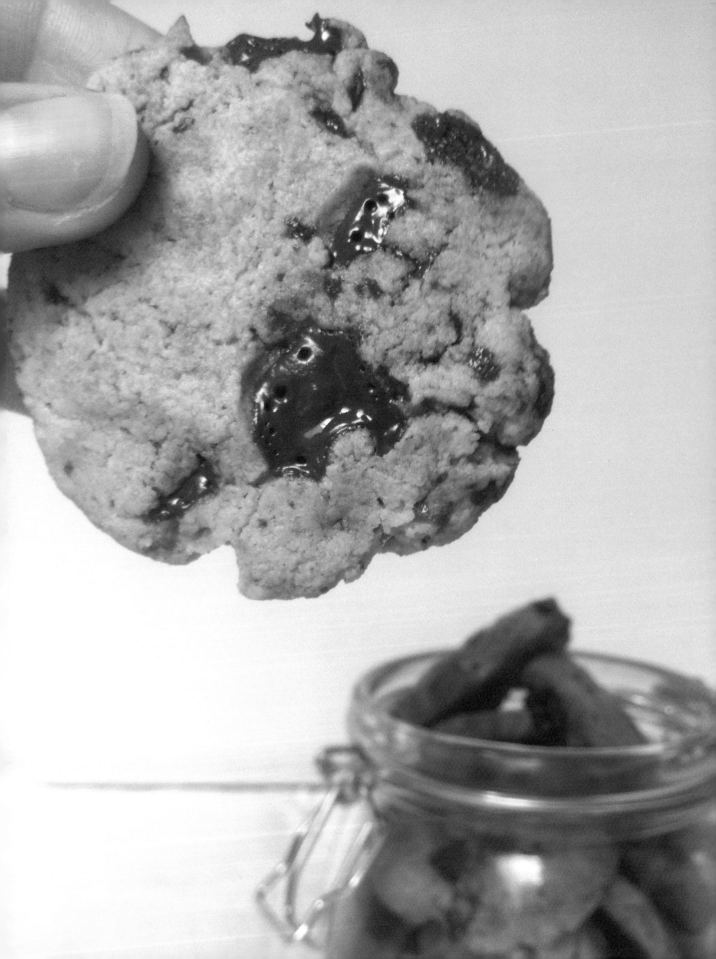

Soft and chewy chocolate chip filled cookies.

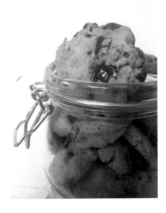

Chocolate chip cookies

- Preheat the oven to 150 degrees celsius (fan assisted oven)

- In a saucepan, heat the dates with a splash of water until softened and can be easily mashed with a fork

- Add the butter (room temperature), dates, bicarbonate of soda and vanilla essence to a blender and blend together until smooth

- Chop the dark chocolate into chunks and stir them into the mixture along with the ground almonds, forming a rough dough

- Tear off small chunks of dough, rolling them into a rough ball shape and gently press down to form your cookies

- Place all the cookies on a sheet of greaseproof paper and place in the oven for approximately 10-15 minutes or until they turn darker brown round the edges

- Remove from the oven and leave to cool on the baking tray

- Once cooled store in a sealed container and hide in a secret place before they all disappear

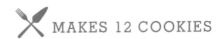 MAKES 12 COOKIES

150g ground almonds

50g butter

50g 70% dark chocolate

¼ teaspoon bicarbonate soda

½ teaspoon vanilla essence

50g dates

147

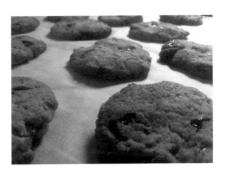

These bites have a soft buttery taste which will keep you coming back for more.

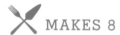 MAKES 8

100g ground almonds

50g butter

50g pecans

½ bicarbonate soda

Pinch salt

1 teaspoon vanilla essence

2 tablespoons honey

148

Buttery pecan bites

- Preheat the oven to 160 degrees celsius (fan assisted oven) and line a baking tray with greaseproof paper

- In a large mixing bowl add the ground almonds, bicarbonate soda, salt, vanilla essence, honey and butter (at room temperature)

- Roughly chop the pecans into chunks and add to the bowl

- Mix together until a rough dough is formed

- Break off pieces of the dough and roll into balls

- Place on the lined baking tray and press down to flatten slightly

- Bake in the oven for 10-15 minutes or until a deeper golden brown

- Remove from the oven and leave to cool

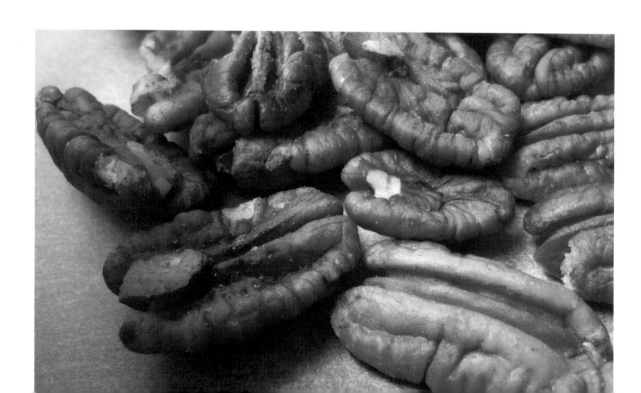

These vanilla pancakes may seem plain but just think of the possibilities! For a sweet kick, serve with fruit and a drizzle of cream. Or add fruits to the mixture, as I've done below, with a pinch of cinnamon and a handful of dried blueberries. Even turn these pancakes into the perfect savoury meal, omitting the honey, vanilla and blueberries. Instead adding a side of sausages, eggs and bacon – English breakfast style.

Vanilla cashew pancakes

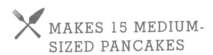

MAKES 15 MEDIUM-SIZED PANCAKES

150g cashews

5 egg whites

1 tablespoon honey

50g butter

½ teaspoon bicarbonate soda

1 teaspoon vanilla essence (optional)

50g dried blueberries (optional)

- Blend the cashews, egg whites, honey, butter and bicarbonate soda in a blender until the mixture is completely smooth and contains no lumps

- Add the dried blueberries and vanilla essence and mix in

- Heat a frying pan on low to medium heat, adding a little butter and splash of oil to the pan to fry the pancakes

- Pour the batter to make little circular pancakes in the frying pan

- Once the pancakes start to puff up and a few bubbles appear on the surface of the pancakes, flip them over and cook on the other side.

- Do this until they are all cooked on both sides and all the batter has been used up

- Serve sweet pancakes with fruit or omit the honey for savoury pancakes

149

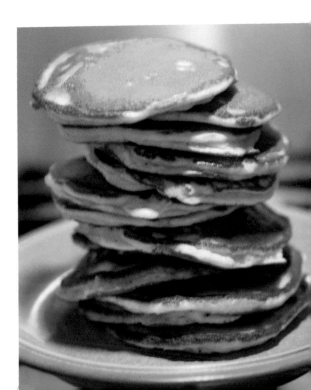

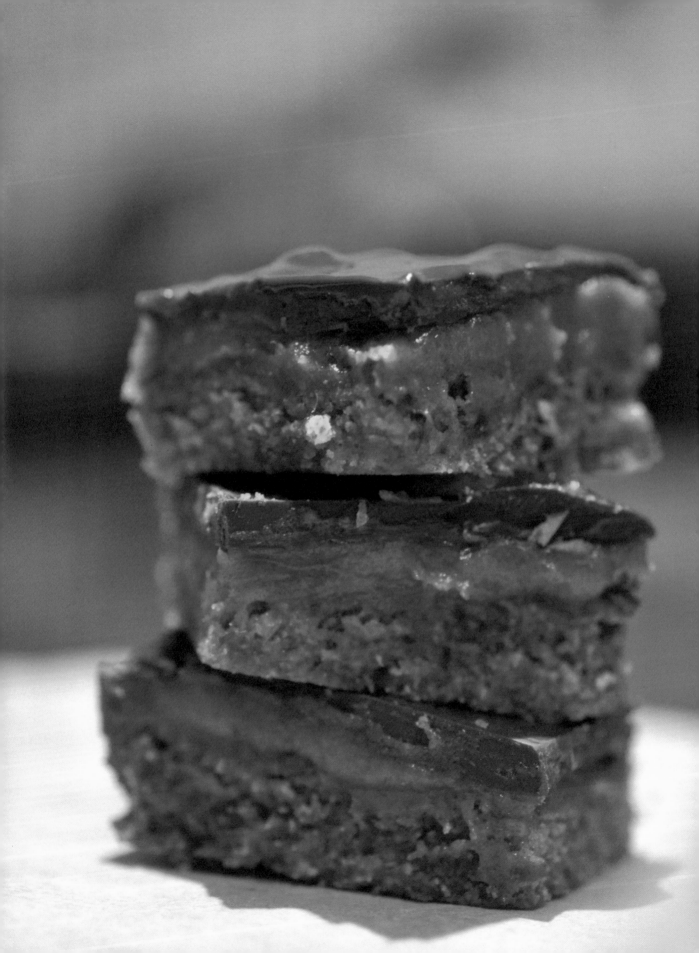

I used to absolutely ADORE millionaire shortbread! There used to be a bakery in Oxford, near where my grandparents lived and whenever I went to stay we would go on a long walk to Headington, always popping in to buy a couple of millionaire shortbread squares. It was all I could do to ward off my uncle back at the house, whom I know shares my adoration for these sweet little squares.

Millionaire shortbread

- Preheat the oven to 150 degrees celsius (fan assisted oven)

- To make the base add the ground almonds, cashew butter, honey, butter and coconut flour into a bowl and mix together until a stiff dough starts to form

- Line a baking tray with greaseproof paper

- Press the dough into a baking tray, giving a thin, even layer of dough, just less than a centimetre thick

- Bake the base in the oven for about 10 minutes or until the base starts to show a bit of colour

- Remove from the oven and leave to cool

- Take one caramel recipe and once the base has cooled, spread a layer over the top of the base and place in the fridge to set

- Break the chocolate into blocks and melt in a glass bowl placed over a small amount of water boiling in a saucepan

- Keep an eye on the temperature and stir the chocolate constantly until all the blocks have melted

- Remove from the heat and leave to cool slightly before spreading the chocolate layer over the top

- Leave to cool and once the chocolate has set, cut into bite size squares

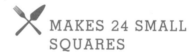

MAKES 24 SMALL SQUARES

Base:

200g ground almonds

2 tablespoons cashew butter

1 tablespoon honey

50g butter

2 tablespoons coconut flour

1 caramel recipe (see tasty toppings)

100g dark chocolate 70%

151

The simple recipe using only 2 ingredients rice and chocolate makes it perfect for a starter recipe for baking with kids. This recipe has the same ideology, using the same small amount of ingredients, just with a healthier kick, swapping the rice for flaked almonds and the more traditional milk chocolate for a darker chocolate.

Crispy cakes

- Heat an inch of water in a saucepan on medium heat, place a bowl in the saucepan so it rests on the edge but does not touch the water in the saucepan.

- Break the chocolate into cubes and place in the bowl to melt

- Stir the chocolate until melted, then remove from the heat

- Place the flaked almonds or chopped pecans and dates into the chocolate and stir in until all the chunks are coated in chocolate

- Place single sweet cases on a plate

- Using two teaspoons, spoon the mixture into the sweet cases

- Place the krispie cakes into the fridge for about an hour to set or until ready to eat

152

These chocolate covered crispy bites have a wonderful contrast of chewy dates and crunchy pecans giving a more distinctive flavour.

Grown-up crispy bites

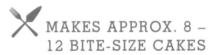 MAKES APPROX. 8 – 12 BITE-SIZE CAKES

50g chopped pecans

25g dates

75g chocolate 70-85%

Kiddie crispy cakes

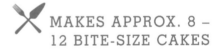 MAKES APPROX. 8 – 12 BITE-SIZE CAKES

50g flaked almonds

50g dark chocolate 70%

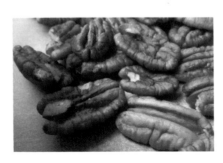

❝ Standing tiptoed in an oversized apron at the kitchen counter, mixing melted chocolate and puffed rice in a large bowl is a childhood pastime few have not experienced. Quick and easy, this two ingredient crispy sweet is a culinary rite of passage. However, you don't have to be a child to enjoy this tradition. ❞

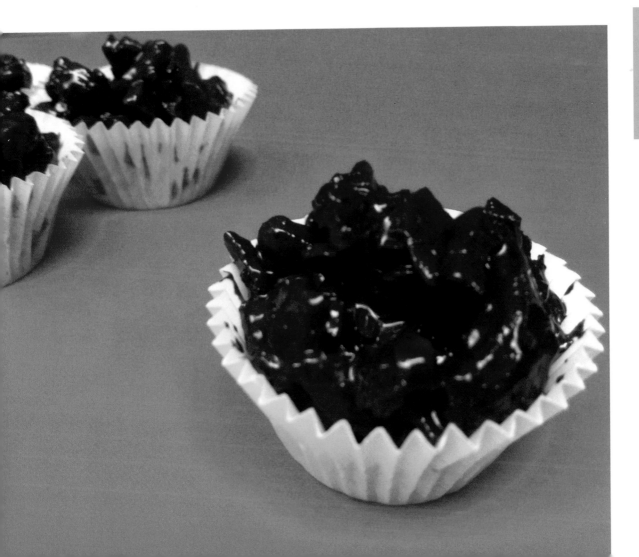

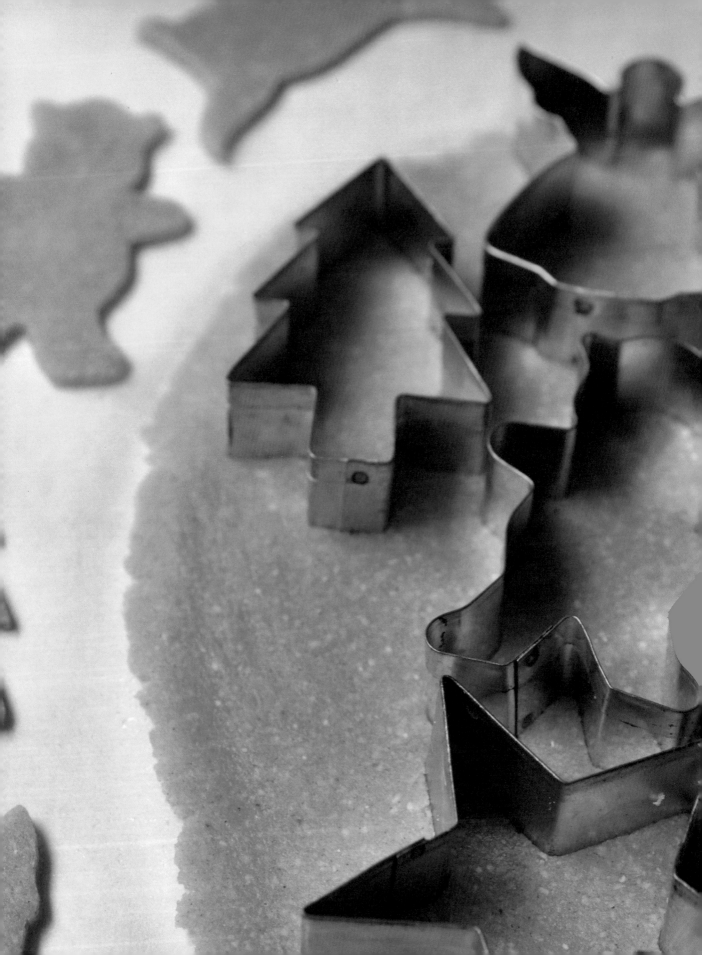

Christmas just wouldn't be complete without rolling out dough surrounded by gingerbread cutters. Then bring these winter spiced characters to life with melted chocolate, pieces of dried fruit and chopped nuts.

Gingerbread men

- Preheat the oven to 160 degrees Celsius (fan assisted oven)

- Mix together all the ingredients

- Use your hands to form a stiff dough

- Sandwich the dough between two sheets of greaseproof paper. This method of rolling out the dough means the dough can be easily rolled out without the use of flour to stop it sticking to the work surface.

- Once the dough has been rolled out to the desired thickness, about ¼ inch, use a gingerbread man biscuit cutter to cut out the individual biscuits

- Use a spatula to move the gingerbread men from the paper onto a greaseproof paper covered baking tray

- Moving the men carefully as they can break apart. If this happens, roll out the dough again, or if the dough has become too warm, place in the fridge for about 20 minutes to cool it down, so it becomes easier to roll out

- Once all the dough has been transformed into gingerbread characters, bake these in the oven for 8-10 minutes or until the edges start turning brown

- Remove from the oven and whilst they are still warm, bring them to life – gently press in chopped nuts, candied nuts, dried fruit pieces or paint on melted chocolate to decorate, giving them eyes, buttons or a cheeky smile.

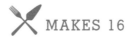 MAKES 16

200g ground almonds

½ teaspoon bicarbonate soda

3 tablespoons honey

25g butter

¼ teaspoon ground mix spice

½ teaspoon cinnamon

2 teaspoons ginger

155

Apple pie

One of my childhood favourites, eat this apple pie warm with a drizzle of single cream.

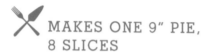

MAKES ONE 9" PIE, 8 SLICES

Pie base:

200g ground almonds

2 tablespoons cashew butter

1 tablespoon honey

50g butter

2 tablespoons coconut flour

Filling:

500g cooking apples

75g butter

Pinch cinnamon

2 tablespoons honey

1 teaspoon vanilla essence

- Preheat the oven to 150 degrees Celsius (fan assisted oven)

- To make the pie base, add the cashew butter, honey, butter and coconut flour to a bowl and mix together, making sure that there are no lumps of coconut flour left

- Add the ground almonds to the mixture and, using your hands, mix together until it forms a sticky dough

- Press the dough into your pie dish, so that it covers the base and sides. It's best to use a pie dish with a removable base for this dish, so it's easier to remove after cooking

- Bake in the oven for 10-15 minutes or until the pie base starts to brown round the edges

- Remove the pie base from the oven and, still in the dish, allow to cool

- To make the filling, chop the cooking apples into thin slices

- Add the honey to a saucepan on low heat

- Stir the honey continuously and after a minute or two the honey will become runny and slowly start to froth

- Watch the honey carefully and as soon as the colour changes to a slightly darker shade, add the butter, vanilla, cinnamon and chopped apples

- Keeping the low heat, stir, coating the apples in the mixture

- Leave this on the heat until the apple pieces are soft

- Once cooked, spread the apple mixture over the base straight away

- Leave to cool until set and you are able to remove from the pie dish or cut into slices

- Eat with a drizzle of cream or to really indulge, a scoop of vanilla ice cream (see blissful bowls)

156

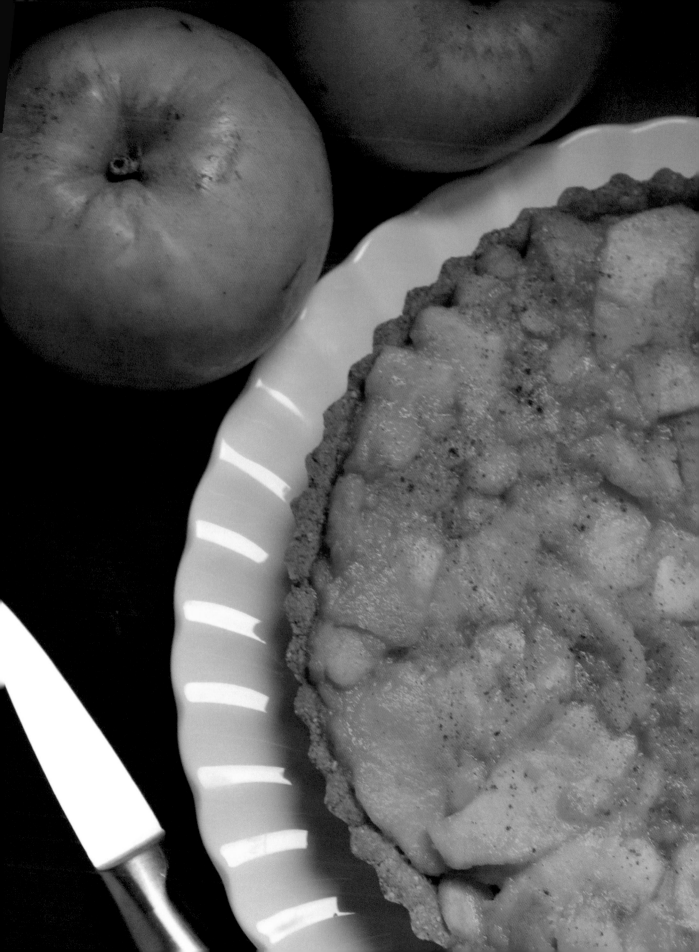

Chocolate coconut pie

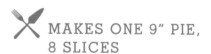

MAKES ONE 9" PIE, 8 SLICES

4 tablespoons almond butter

200g ground almonds

50g butter

100g dates

Chocolate filling:

100g coconut block

200ml water

75g dates

2½ tablespoon cocoa powder

1 teaspoon vanilla essence

158

- To make the pie base, blend together the almond butter, dates and butter – I use a hand blender but you could use any type of blender

- Add the ground almonds to the mixture and mix together until it forms a dough

- I always use a pie dish with a removable base for ease of removal. However, if you don't have one, you can always place a layer of cling film over the pie dish before pressing the dough into your pie dish, so that it covers the base and sides

- Put the pie base in the fridge to set, whilst you make the filling

- To make the filling, add the coconut to a saucepan on low heat

- When this begins to melt, add the water and stir until the coconut melts into the water

- Add the dates, cocoa powder and vanilla essence and stir until the dates become softer

- Blend the ingredients in the saucepan until the mixture forms a smooth consistency, with no lumps

- Allow the mixture to cool before pouring into the pie base, then return to the fridge

- Once the mixture and pie base have completely set, the pie can be removed from the dish and sliced

- Keep the pie in the fridge to keep it cool if any slices are left over

- I sometimes get too impatient and pop it in the freezer to let it set quicker – sometimes you just need an immediate chocolate hit

This no bake pie makes for a wonderful cold dessert with a smooth chocolate filling.

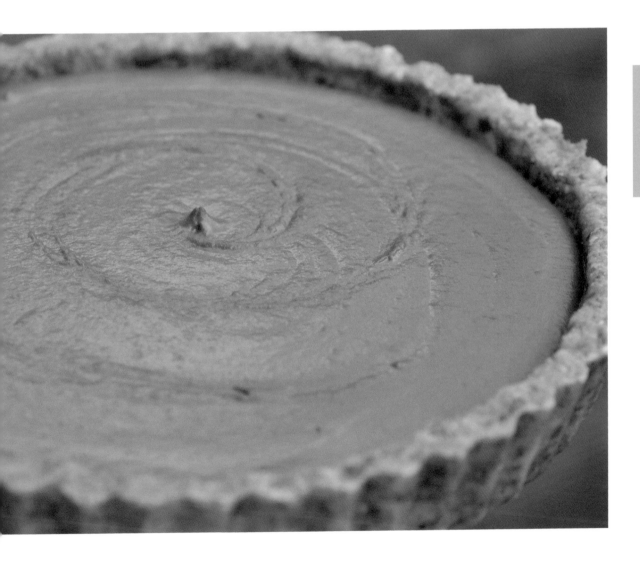

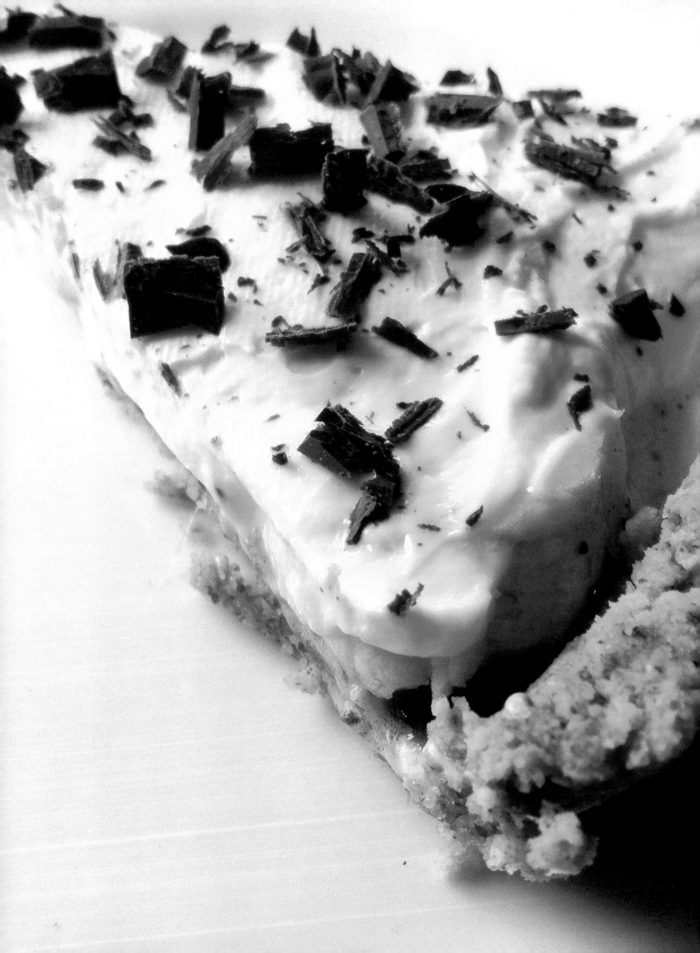

Banoffee pie

- Preheat the oven to 150 degrees Celsius (fan assisted oven)

- To make the pie base, blend together the almond butter, dates and butter – I use a hand blender

- Add the ground almonds to the mixture and mix together until it forms a dough

- Press the dough into a pie dish, so that it covers the base and sides

- Bake the pie base in the oven for 10-15 minutes, and get started on the filling

- To make the filling, add the dates and the water to a saucepan on low heat

- When the dates begin to soften, add the butter and cream and remove from the heat

- Blend the mixture together until the caramel has a smooth and thick consistency

- Put aside to cool

- Remove the pie base from the oven, once turning brown round the edges, and leave to cool

- Once cooled, spread the caramel over the pie base

- Chop the bananas into slices, adding them on top of the caramel layer

- Whisk the cream until stiff peaks appear

- Spoon the cream over the top of the pie, until the top is completely covered

- Grate the dark chocolate over the top to finish

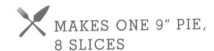 MAKES ONE 9″ PIE, 8 SLICES

Base:

4 tablespoons almond butter

200g ground almonds

50g butter

100g dates

1 thick caramel recipe

2 bananas

A few blocks 70% dark chocolate

Whipped cream

161

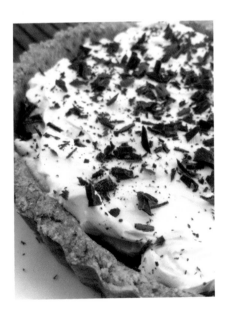

Dates and banana give the natural sweetness in this pie.

*❛ When summer comes around I love these cute little tarts.
As a child I would stay with my grandparents during the summer.
Going to local pick-your own farms was an annual tradition,
always returning with baskets full of the colourful fruits.
This recipe makes the most of juicy seasonal berries in perfect
combination with cream and a flaky pastry case. ❜*

Summer berry tarts

✕ MAKES 6 4″ TARTS

Pie bases:

200g ground almonds

2 tablespoons cashew butter

1 tablespoon honey

50g butter

2 tablespoon coconut flour

Single cream

A handful each of:

Strawberries

Raspberries

Blueberries

Blackberries

- Preheat the oven to 150 degrees Celsius (fan assisted oven)

- To make the pie bases, add the cashew butter, honey, butter and coconut flour to a bowl and mix together, making sure that there are no lumps of coconut flour left

- Add the ground almonds to the mixture and, using your hands, mix together until it forms a sticky dough

- Press the dough into individual pie dishes, so that it covers the base and sides. It's best to use individual pie dishes with removable bases for this dish, so it's easier to remove after cooking

- Bake in the oven for 10-15 minutes or until the pie base starts to brown round the edges

- Remove the pie bases from the oven and allow to cool before removing from the pie dishes

- Chop the strawberries and wash all the berries

- Add the berries to the pie base

- Pour the single cream over the top of the berries

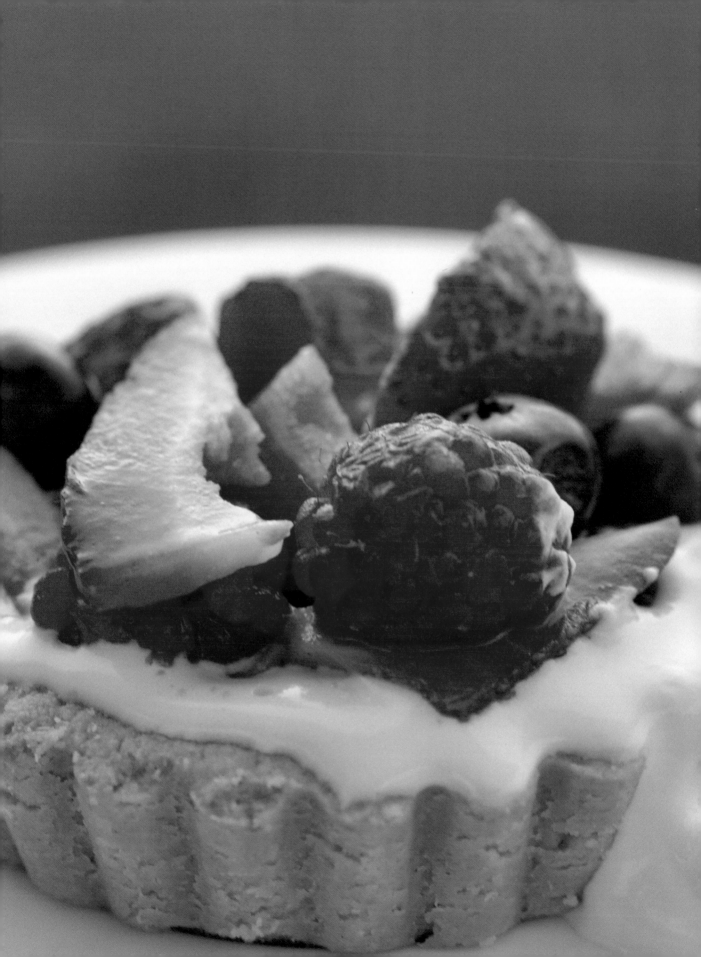

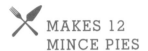

**MAKES 12
MINCE PIES**

Pastry makes 12 pie cases:

100g ground almonds

1 tablespoon coconut flour

1 tablespoon cashew butter

25g coconut butter

1 tablespoon honey

Filling makes enough for 12
mince pies and a little more to
set aside:

250g peeled cooking apples

Zest and juice of 1 lemon

Zest and juice of one
clementine

1 tablespoon honey

2 teaspoons ground mixed
spice

¼ teaspoon cinnamon

100g raisins

100g sultanas

100g currants

Pinch salt

½ teaspoon vanilla essence

75g suet

2 tablespoons brandy

Festive mince pies

Filling:

- Preheat 140 degrees celsius (fan assisted oven)

- Peel and chop approximately 1-2 cooking apples to make 250g

- Finely chop the apple and place in a large baking dish along with the rest of the filling ingredients and mix together

- Cover the baking dish with tin foil and place in the oven for an hour

- After an hour, give the mixture a stir and place back in the oven for another hour or until the mincemeat is cooked through and the apples are able to be easily mashed with a fork

- Once cooked through, remove from the oven, uncover the foil and leave to cool

An absolute must for Christmas cuisine. Christmas food tends to be a time of year for alcohol drenched puddings and as much chocolate and sweets as you can manage. With flaky pastry cases, these mince pies mimick the traditional little pies, found everywhere around Christmas time. These fruity mincemeat packed mini pies use the fruits natural sweetness with a tablespoon of honey added to give them a deep sweet honey spiced flavour.

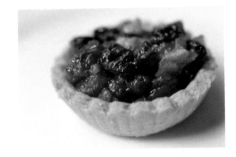

Cases:

- Whilst the mincemeat filling is cooking, start making the cases

- In a mixing bowl, add the ground almonds, coconut flour, honey, cashew butter and coconut butter. Use the coconut butter at room temperature so it is soft enough to mix in.

- Mix together until it forms a dough

- Then sandwich the dough between two pieces of greaseproof paper and roll out till the sheet of pastry is approximately 3 to 4 millimetres thick

- Use a circular, fluted biscuit cutter and cut out little circular discs

- Line a cupcake tray with cupcake cases or mince pie cases

- Using a spatula, carefully move the circular pastry discs from the greaseproof paper and place them into the cupcake cases

- Once the mincemeat has been removed from the oven, turn the temperature up to 150 degrees celsius (fan assisted oven)

- These pie cases cook extremely quickly and so should only take approximately 5-10 minutes so keep a close eye whilst baking so they don't burn

- Once turning slightly golden brown, remove from the oven and leave to cool

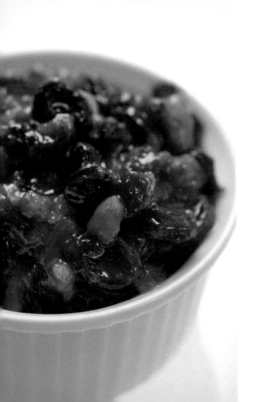

Mince pies:

- Simply spoon the mincemeat into the pie cases until all the mince pies are filled

- Eat on their own or with the topping of your choice and if you can bear to spare one, leave one out on the mantelpiece with a carrot on Christmas eve

165

Lucy's waffles

- Preheat a waffle maker

- Mix all ingredients together in a large mixing bowl until all the ingredients are combined

- Once the waffle maker is heated, add the mixture to the waffle maker and follow your waffle makers instructions

- Once the waffles have finished cooking, remove carefully from the waffle maker and serve hot or cold, plain, or with your choice of toppings

✗ MAKES 4 WAFFLES

4 egg whites

40ml milk

½ teaspoon bicarbonate soda

100g ground almonds

3 tablespoons honey

166

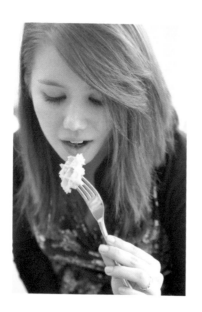

Now. I aimed to sing these waffles praises, telling you how thick they are and comforting when served warm with ice cream, but after making these for the first time, I'll never regret making anything more. The minute these hit the plate, with the smell wafting out of the door, I had doomed myself. My sister, Lucy, is the most difficult person to cook for. She has very simple tastes and doesn't like fussy foods with strong flavours. So my hopes weren't high for when she came down to see what was on offer. She took a waffle, suspiciously sniffed at it (she knows my tendency to put unusual ingredients in everything) before cautiously taking a bite. By the time I turned around and was ready to get a plate for my taste test, I reached for a waffle, to find one left, with Lucy's fork hovering expectantly over it. Since then, I have not had a minute's peace. Not a day passes when I don't get a request for these waffles. I keep thinking she'll tire of them but unfortunately, she hasn't yet (I'll let you know if she ever does).

So be warned. Everyone loves wonderful, thick waffles but just know that there's always the possibility you might be making these for weeks...

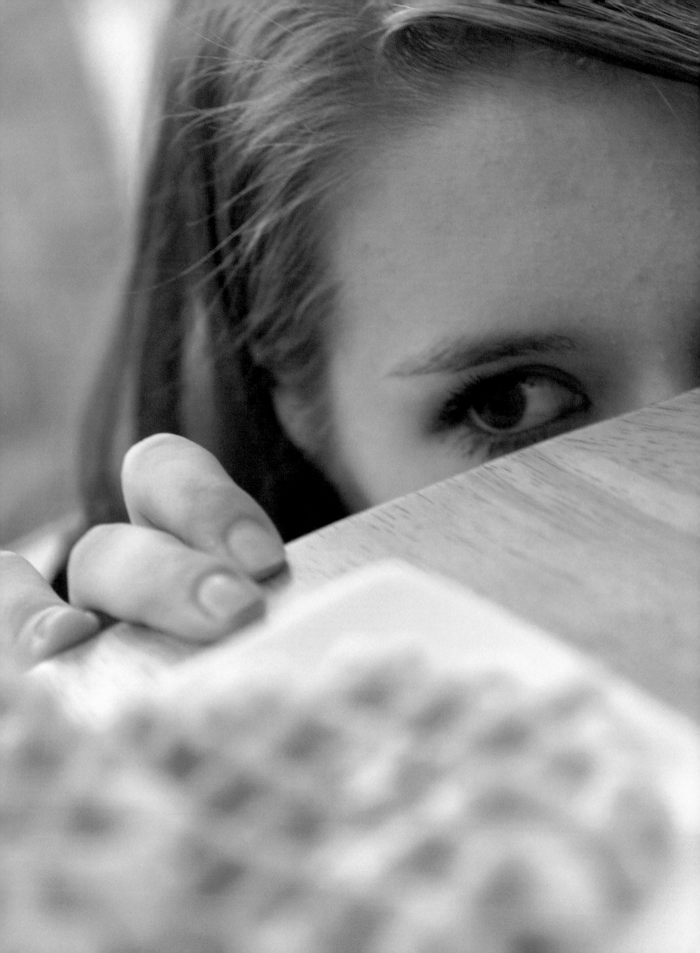

I DON'T KNOW WHAT IT IS BUT ANYTHING
SERVED IN A BOWL IS PARAMOUNT WHEN
IT COMES TO COMFORT FOOD. HUDDLING
OVER A BOWL OF CRUMBLE SMOTHERED IN
CUSTARD ON A COLD WINTER'S NIGHT OR
A REFRESHINGLY COLD BOWL OF SORBET
OR ICE CREAM ON A HOT SUMMER'S DAY.
THEN OF COURSE THERE ARE THE STAPLES;
WAITING TO START THE DAY WITH A MORNING
BOWL OF FRUIT TOPPED WITH GRANOLA AND
A TABLESPOON OF CRÈME FRAICHE. THERE'S
A BOWL FOR EVERY OCCASION

blissful bowls

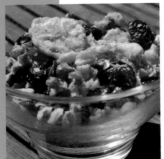

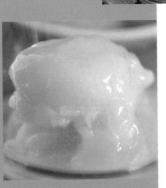

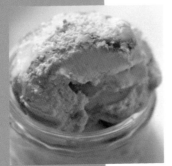

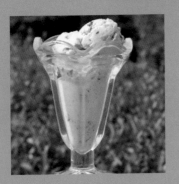

169

Muesli

- Preheat the oven to 160 degrees celsius (fan assisted oven)

- Chop the walnuts and dates into small chunks

- Add all the ingredients in the bowl and mix together

- Line a baking tray with greaseproof paper and spread out the mixture over the baking tray

- Crisp in the oven for about 15 minutes or until the muesli takes on a bit of colour

- Remove from the oven and leave to cool

- Store in a jar or a sealable plastic bag to keep the muesli fresh

- Serve with chopped fruit and crème fraiche or with a good splash of milk

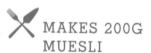

MAKES 200G MUESLI

75g flaked almonds

50g walnuts

25g pumpkin seeds

3 tablespoons olive oil

½ teaspoon vanilla essence

Large pinch cinnamon

50g dates

170

Chopped dates give this otherwise savoury muesli an occasional sweet bite.

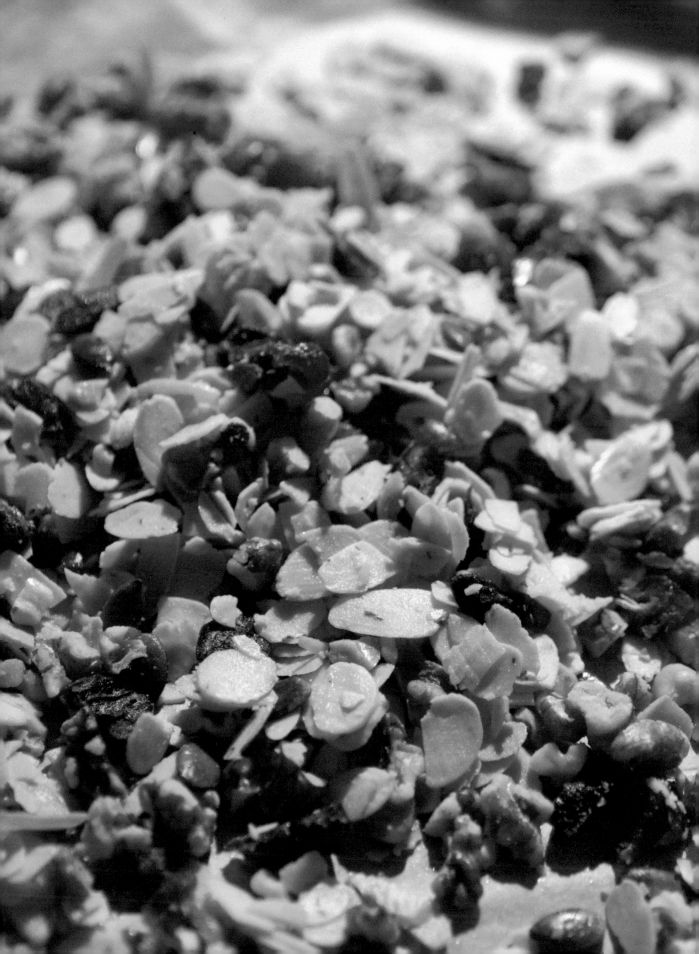

I've always been a bit of a cereal addict. It's the crunch that gets me. A few slices of pear or melon and a few red grapes with a handful of granola and a splash of milk over the top give a crunchy fruit and nut start to the day.

Sunny granola

✕ MAKES 250G GRANOLA

25g banana coins

25g dried cranberries

50g brazil nuts

50g pecans

50g walnuts

50g desiccated coconut

2 tablespoons walnut oil

1 tablespoon honey

- Preheat the oven to 160 degrees celsius (fan assisted oven)
- Chop the brazil nuts, banana coins, pecans and walnuts into small chunks
- Add all the ingredients in the bowl and mix together
- Line a baking tray with greaseproof paper and spread out the mixture over the baking tray
- Crisp in the oven for about 15 minutes or until the granola takes on a bit of colour
- Remove from the oven and leave to cool
- Store in a jar or container or a sealable plastic bag to keep the granola fresh
- Serve with fresh fruit or milk

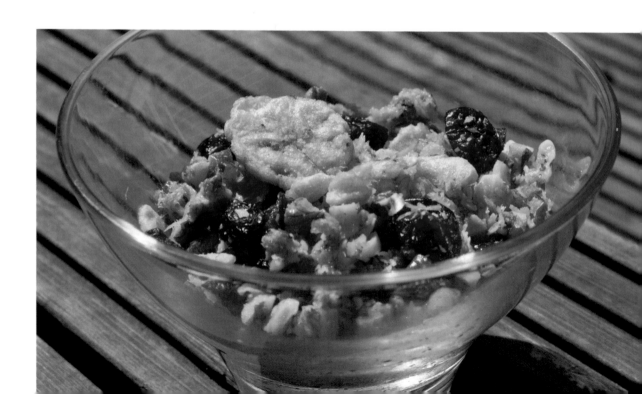

Wonderfully warm, this breakfast wins my heart on a cold winter morning.

Cold morning porridge

- Use a blender or a grinder attachment for a hand blender, pulsing until the cashews reach a coarse flour consistency – it's best to pulse the cashews so you do not over blend and end up with nut butter

- Whisk together the egg whites and water and pour into a saucepan along with the cashews, vanilla, salt, cinnamon , butter, coconut flour and honey

- Place the saucepan over a low to medium heat and stir continuously

- The mixture will begin to thicken, keep stirring over the heat until the porridge reaches the thickness you want

- Serve in a bowl whilst still hot and drizzle with honey

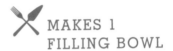

MAKES 1 FILLING BOWL

25g cashews

2½ level tablespoons coconut flour

2 egg whites

250ml water

Splash vanilla essence

Pinch sea salt

1 tablespoon honey

1 teaspoon butter

Large pinch cinnamon

173

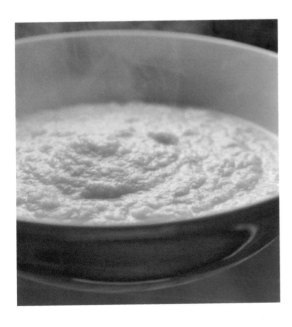

Totally refreshing and made with only two ingredients, it really couldn't be more simple!

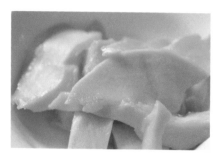

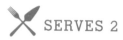 SERVES 2

300g mango

250ml water

174

Mango sorbet

- Cut, peel and weigh out the mango

- Blend the mango and water in a blender until a smooth, viscous consistency is reached

- Pour the mixture into an ice cream maker and follow the ice cream makers instructions

- Once the sorbet is frozen to the desired consistency, scoop out of the ice cream maker and either serve immediately or store in a sealed container in the freezer

- When defrosting later, remove from the freezer and leave out until scoopable. Alternatively, heat in the microwave for a few seconds

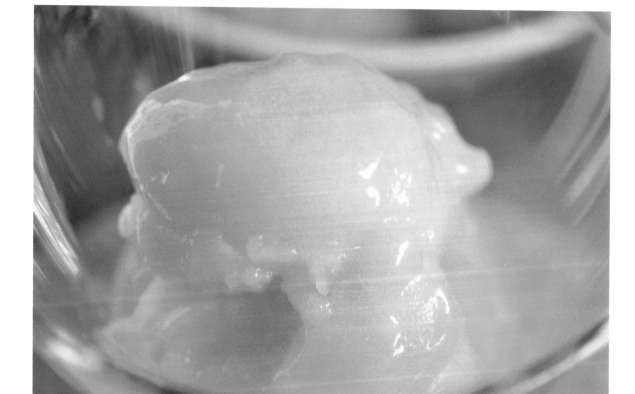

Pear crumble

- Preheat the oven to 150 degrees celsius (fan assisted oven)

- To prepare the pear base, peel the pears and chop into slices

- Add the pears, vanilla essence, water and cinnamon to a small saucepan on a low heat

- Leave the pears to simmer, occasionally stirring the pear slices

- Whilst waiting for the pears to cook, prepare the topping by adding the ground almonds, flaked almonds, butter, vanilla essence, cinnamon and honey to a bowl

- Using your hands, rub the mixture together on the tips of your fingers, causing the mixture to literally, crumble

- Once the pears are soft enough to easily cut, take them off the heat and spoon the pears into a small casserole dish (approx. 18cm by 12cm), covering the entire base

- Sprinkle the topping over the pears

- Place the crumble in the oven for 30-40 minutes or until the top shows some colour and starts to brown

- Remove the dish from the oven and serve immediately whilst still hot, ideally with a large scoop of vanilla ice cream

Crumble is such a comforting dessert. Essentially coupled with custard or a scoop of ice cream. Trust me.

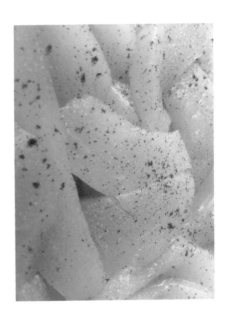

175

✕ SERVES 2

3 large pears

¼ teaspoon vanilla essence

Large pinch cinnamon

1 tablespoon water

Topping;

200g ground almonds

50g flaked almonds

50g butter

½ teaspoon vanilla essence

Pinch cinnamon

1 tablespoon honey

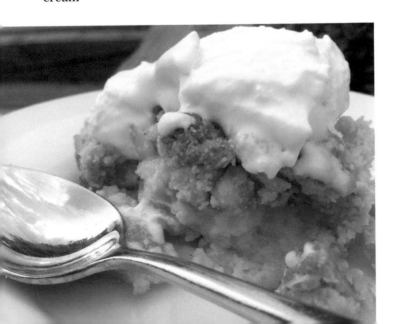

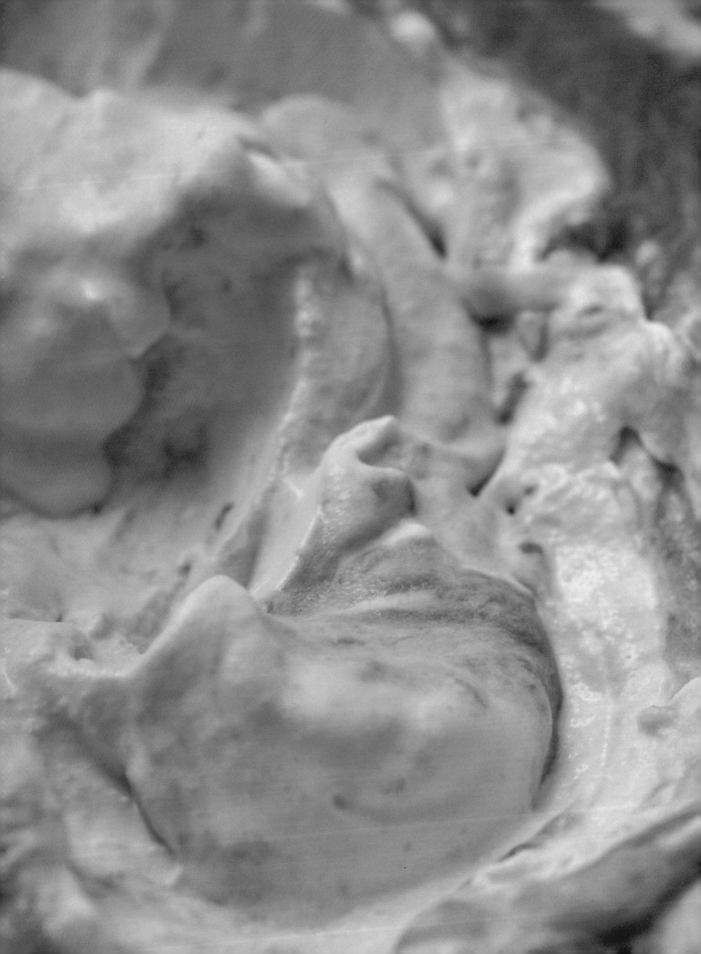

Raspberry ripple ice cream

Make the ice cream:

- Add all the ice cream ingredients and blend until a smooth consistency is reached

- Add the mixture to the ice cream maker and follow the ice cream makers instructions

Make the raspberry-strawberry couli:

- Add the raspberries and strawberries to a small saucepan on a low to medium heat, occasionally stirring

- As the berries begin to break down, stir in the butter and honey, continuing to stir and simmer on a low heat

- Once the berries have completely broken down, pass the mixture through a sieve to remove the seeds

- Leave the sieved coulis to cool

- Once the ice cream reaches a thick consistency, spoon the ice cream into a sealable container

- Pour the coulis over the ice cream and roughly swirl into the vanilla ice cream, making ripples of fruit throughout the ice cream

- Place the ice cream container in the freezer for approximately an hour or until the ice cream completely sets

- Remove from the freezer and leave at room temperature until scoopable and serve

Here you find the combined effort from mother Whiteley and myself. Suddenly announcing a craving for raspberry ripple ice cream (with no particular previous penchant for this particular flavour) we had to come up with something quickly. We made a batch of my original vanilla ice cream and swirled in my fruity raspberry and strawberry couli. Craving managed!

177

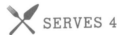 SERVES 4

Original vanilla ice cream:

3 tablespoon cashew butter

300ml milk

600ml cream

1½ teaspoons vanilla essence

2 tablespoons honey

Raspberry-Strawberry couli:

400g raspberries

200g strawberries

50g butter

2 tablespoons honey

Soft vanilla ice cream; cool and refreshing as a stand alone dessert or a beautiful addition to a helping of warm crumble or a slice of pie.

Sweet and simple vanilla ice cream

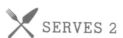

SERVES 2

150ml milk

300ml cream

2 tablespoons honey

1 teaspoon vanilla essence

A few cubes of dark chocolate (optional)

178

- Simply mix the first four ingredients in a bowl – you may need to use a blender to ensure the honey is incorporated and does not just sink to the bottom of the bowl

- Add to your ice cream maker and follow your ice cream makers instructions

- Once frozen to the desired consistency – this should make a very soft creamy scoop – serve immediately with the dark chocolate grated over the top or store in a sealed container in the freezer

- When defrosting later, remove from the freezer and leave out until scoopable. Alternatively, heat in the microwave for a few seconds, keep an eye open as it defrosts or you may find yourself with ice cream soup

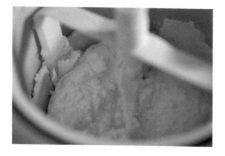

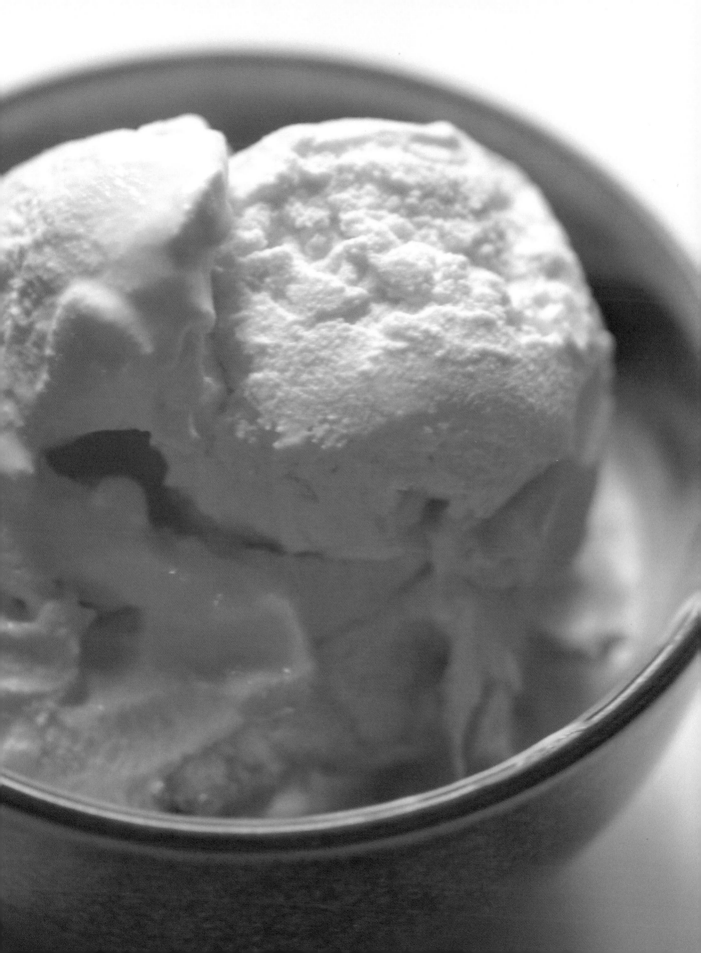

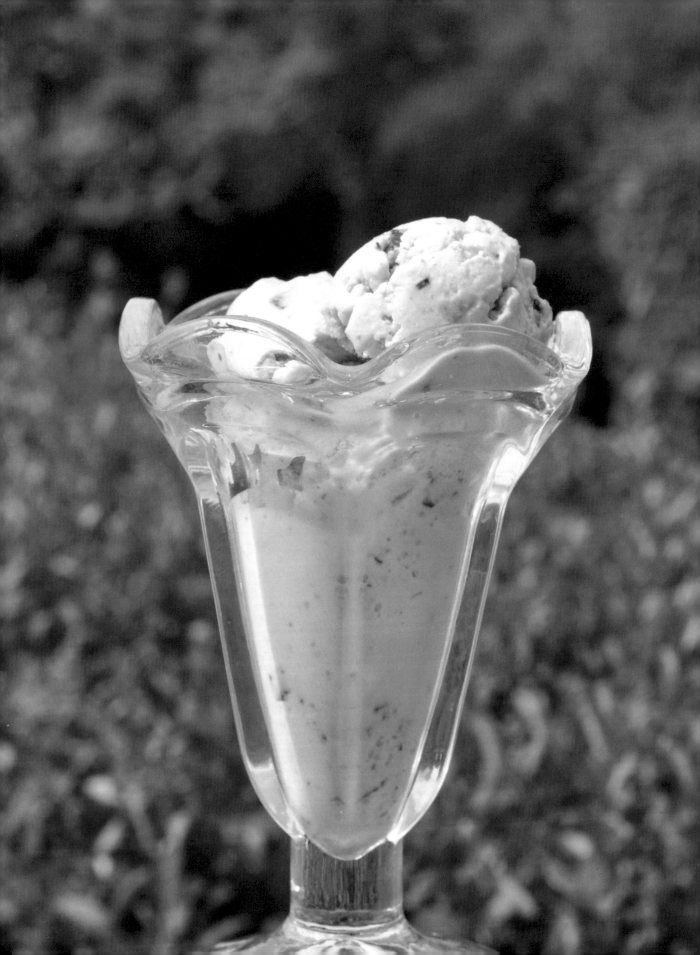

Dairy free? I could definitely not let you miss out on ice cream. Using creamy roasted cashew butter and adding chocolate chips, this ice cream has a distinctive nutty taste, definitely an individual choc-chip ice cream.

Dairy free choc chip, cashew ice cream

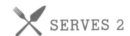 SERVES 2

- Blend together the cashew butter, water, vanilla essence and honey until smooth

- Pour the mixture into an ice cream maker and freeze according to your ice cream makers instructions

- Once the ice cream is done, serve immediately or place in a covered container in the freezer

- Before serving ice cream after freezing, remove from the freezer and leave out until scoopable. Alternatively, place in the microwave for a few seconds, to soften

5 tablespoons cashew butter

250ml water

½ teaspoon vanilla essence

1 tablespoon honey

50g dark chocolate (optional)

181

I keep a jar of my crumbly pecan topping (see tasty toppings) close at hand for rushed mornings when a quick breakfast is essential.

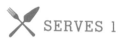

SERVES 1

Breakfast bowl

4 heaped tablespoons half fat crème fraiche

½ banana

1 small handful Crumbly pecan topping

- Add the crème fraiche to a bowl
- Slice the banana into the bowl
- Add a small handful of the topping
- Stir together and dig in!

182

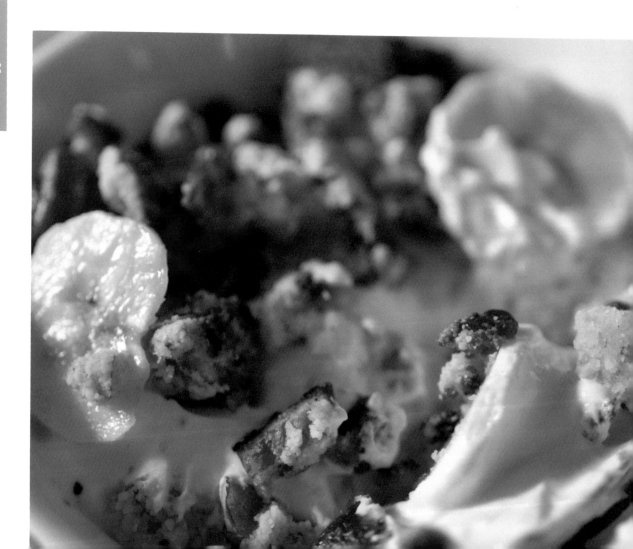

Smooth chocolaty dairy free pudding. For the best results use a high speed blender to end up with a silky smooth pudding.

Chocolate pudding

- Heat the dates with a splash of water in a saucepan until soft

- Blend together the dates, cashews, cocoa and water using a blender

- Spoon the mousse in to a bowl and place in the fridge

- Once cooled, spoon into small individual bowls and serve

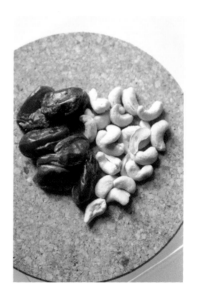

183

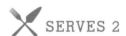

SERVES 2

3 tablespoons cocoa powder

50g dates

50g cashew nuts

100ml water

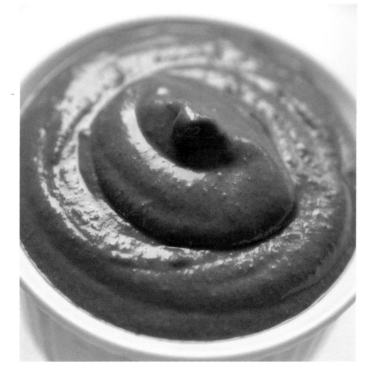

THERE ARE TIMES WHEN A MEAL IS JUST
TOO HEAVY. WHAT WOULD REALLY HIT THE
SPOT IS A LIGHT, REFRESHING DRINK.
SURPRISINGLY FILLING, SIPPING ON
WHOLESOME, NUTRIENT PACKED DRINKS
CAN BE A QUICK AND EASY ALTERNATIVE
TO A BULKY MEAL

delicious drinks

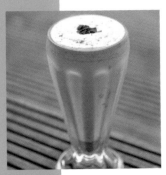

185

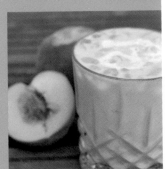

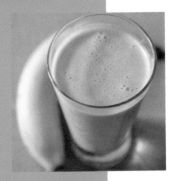

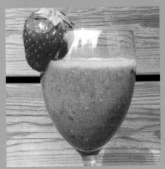

Walking through town there used to be a gorgeous milkshake shop whipping up milkshakes from your chosen ice cream flavour. For me it was mint chocolate chip every time. Nothing would beat the fresh minty taste with scattered crunchy chocolate pieces.

Minty, chocolate shake

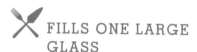

FILLS ONE LARGE GLASS

100ml cream

1 tablespoon peppermint essence

200ml crushed ice

50g dark chocolate

1 teaspoon honey

50ml water

186

- Add the cream, peppermint essence, honey and water to a blender and blend until mixed

- Add the crushed ice and once again blend until the mixture thickens

- Break the dark chocolate into cubes and add to the blender

- Pulse the mixture to produce finely chopped chocolate chunks throughout the mixture

- Pour the mixture into glasses and drink immediately

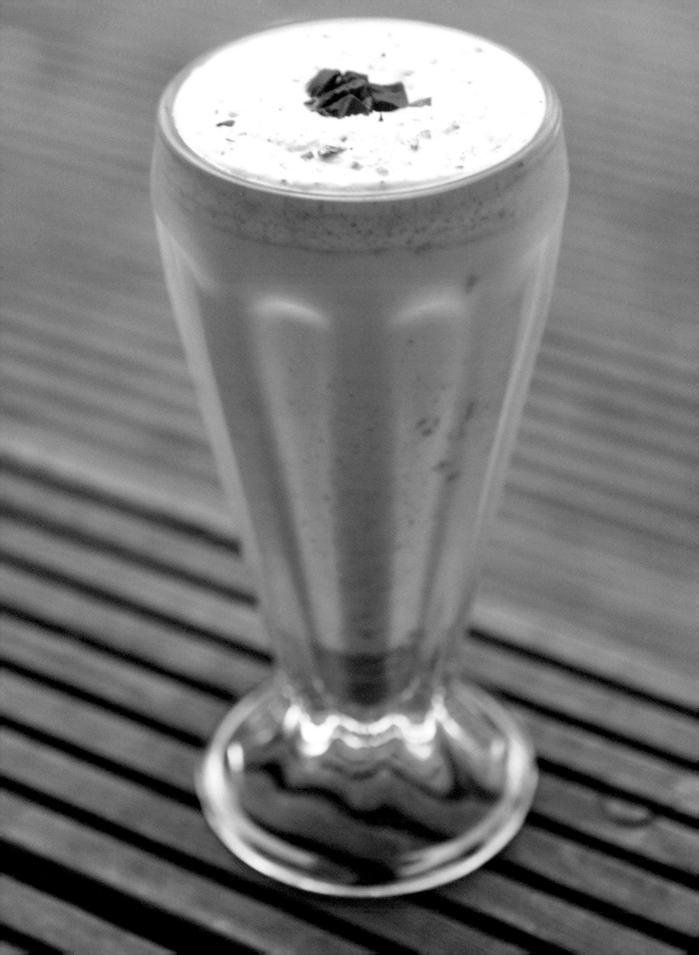

❛ Lightly flavoured, refreshing drink for hot summer days. Feel free to add more lemon juice and honey to increase the flavour and sweetness of the drink. ❜

Lemonade

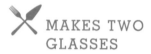 MAKES TWO GLASSES

50ml lemon juice

300ml sparkling water

1½ tablespoons honey

Large pinch of salt

- Mix all the ingredients in a serving jug until all ingredients are incorporated – be sure to mix the honey in, as sometimes it can sink to the bottom of the jug

- Place jug on the table along with serving glasses

❛ Smooth creamy hot chocolate. Make with milk or for a dairy free version use either coconut milk or cashew milk. ❜

Hot chocolate

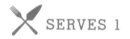 SERVES 1

200ml milk

2 tablespoons cocoa powder

1 tablespoon honey

Pinch salt

Few drops vanilla essence

- Add the milk to a small saucepan and simmer on a low heat

- Mix in the cocoa, honey, salt and vanilla essence to the milk and continue to heat until the mixture begins to bubble

- Remove from the heat and pour into a mug to serve

188

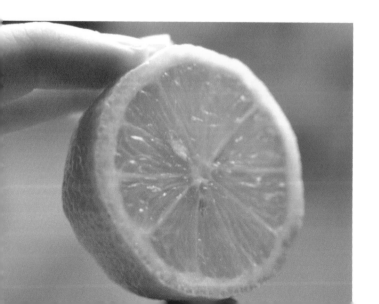

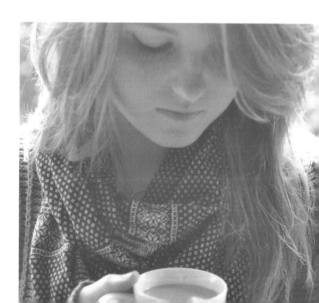

Decadent chocolate milkshake

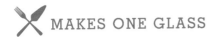 **MAKES ONE GLASS**

100g vanilla ice cream (see recipes in blissful bowls)

80ml milk

1½ tablespoons cocoa powder

1 teaspoon honey

Pinch sea salt

- Place all ingredients in a blender and blend
- Pour into a glass and top with an additional scoop of ice cream
- Drink immediately

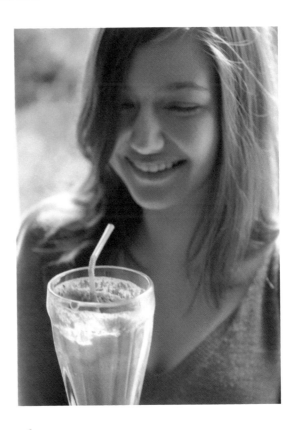

❛ *Definitely a decadent treat, summer would come round and my mum would get out the blender and vanilla ice cream. This could mean only one thing. Chocolate ice cream milk shake! She would then blend together the ingredients, and in seconds she would be pouring the thick creamy drink into glasses for my sisters and I. With an extra scoop of vanilla ice cream floating on top, resistance was futile. Sipping our milkshakes through coloured straws whilst squealing how good it tasted, coupled with smeared chocolate smiles, savouring every sip. This shake never fails to rekindle that childish excitement, always leaving me with a chocolate smile.* ❜

Creamy but fresh and light, perfect for sipping on whilst relaxing in the garden.

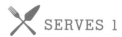 SERVES 1

2 peaches

100ml water

Crushed ice

4 tablespoons single cream

1 tablespoon lemon juice

Peach cooler

- Slice the peaches and add to the blender along with the water, 3 tablespoons single cream and lemon juice until smooth

- Add the crushed ice to a glass and pour the peach drink over the ice

- To serve, swirl the final tablespoon of cream over the top of the drink

190

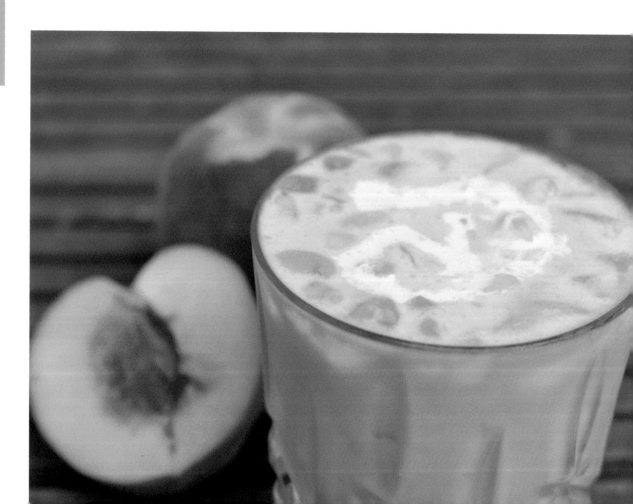

Peanut banana smoothie

- Add all ingredients to a blender and blend until smooth
- Pour into a glass and serve

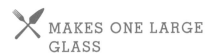

MAKES ONE LARGE GLASS

3 tablespoons peanut butter

100g banana

100ml water

Pinch cinnamon

Pinch sea salt

50ml milk

191

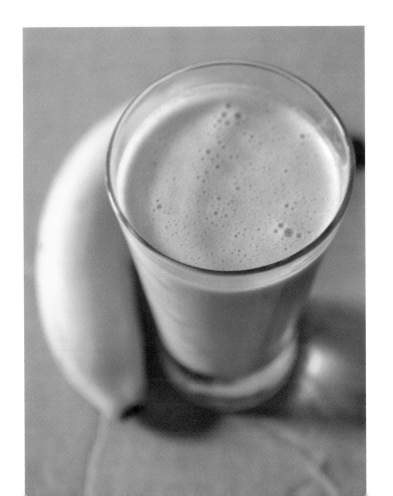

An easy source of nutrition, this smoothie is packed with energy to keep you going throughout the day.

Melon and strawberry smoothie

✗ MAKES 2 LARGE GLASSES

½ honeydew melon

300g strawberries

1 tablespoon lemon juice

Pinch sea salt

100ml half fat crème fraiche

- Wash and prepare the strawberries and melon and add to a blender along with the other ingredients and blend until smooth

- Pour into glasses, add a few ice cubes and serve

This drink is yet another result of countless wanderings through town. During summer, I would wear myself out, throwing myself into athletics practise, afterwards passing by a fruit smoothie shop to grab a tall drink of melon and strawberry smoothie.